Current Topics in Extrapyramidal Disorders

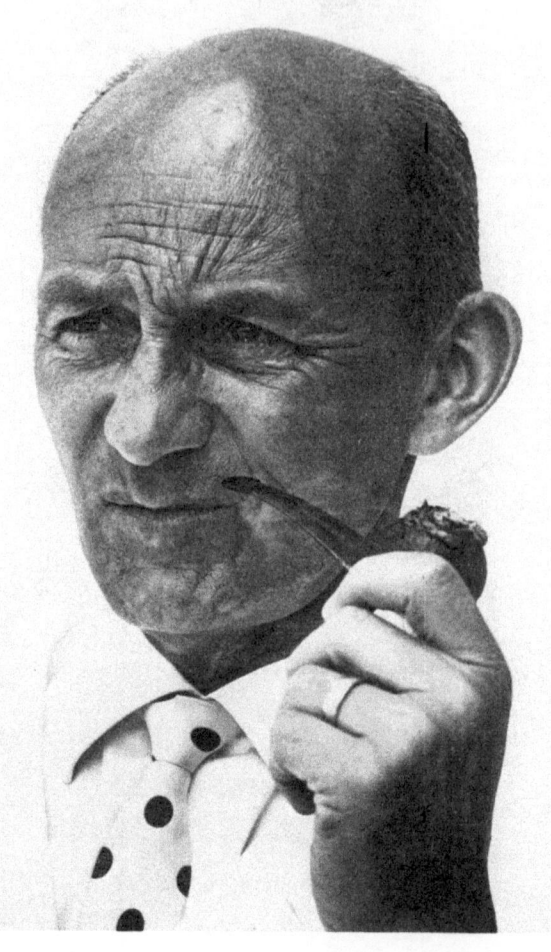

Journal of Neural Transmission
Supplementum 16

Current Topics in Extrapyramidal Disorders

**Edited by A. Carlsson,
K. Jellinger, and P. Riederer**

Springer-Verlag
Wien New York

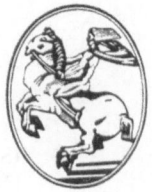

Prof. Dr. Arvid Carlsson
Department of Pharmacology, University of Göteborg, Göteborg, Sweden

Prof. Dr. Kurt Jellinger
Ludwig Boltzmann-Institut für Klinische Neurobiologie und
Neurologische Abteilung, Krankenhaus der Stadt Wien-Lainz, Wien, Austria

Doz. Dr. Peter Riederer
Ludwig Boltzmann-Institut für Klinische Neurobiologie
Krankenhaus der Stadt Wien-Lainz, Wien, Austria

With 1 Portrait and 31 Figures

Library of Congress Cataloging in Publication Data. Main entry under title: Current topics in extrapyramidal disorders. (Journal of neural transmission : Supplementum ; 16.) 1. Extrapyramidal tracts—Diseases. 2. Parkinsonism. 3. Movement disorders. I. Carlsson, Arvid. II. Jellinger, Kurt. III. Riederer, Peter, 1942—. IV. Series. [DNLM: 1. Basal ganglia diseases. 2. Parkinson's disease. 3. Antiparkinson agents. W1 J0781A no. 16 / WL307 C976.] RC361.C92. 616.8'3. 80-11898

ISSN 0303-6995
ISBN-13:978-3-7091-8584-1   e-ISBN-13:978-3-7091-8582-7
DOI: 10.1007/978-3-7091-8582-7

Preface

The scientific work of Walther Birkmayer is grounded on his ability to turn what was often a mass of clinical details into the basis for a hypothesis for a new therapeutic approach toward solving the problems of a patient's illness.

Birkmayer first became known when, during the Second World War, he built up a clinic for brain injuries in Vienna, in which over 3000 patients were treated. The study of changes in the autonomic functions of the nervous system in these patients as well as the problems of rehabilitation were published in a monograph, "Hirn-verletzungen". Consequently, this was his major scientific interest during the post-war years. His book, "Klinik und Therapie der vegetativen Funktionsstörungen" published with W. Winkler, brought Birkmayer recognition in the German-speaking world.

In 1954 he took over the Neurological Department of the Geriatric Hospital of Vienna in Lainz, where he remained until his retirement in 1975.

International acclaim followed his breakthrough with the clinical application of L-DOPA in Parkinson's disease. Birkmayer, as a strong adherent to the scientific interpretation of neurological and psychiatric disease, has encouraged multidisciplinary research. This is reflected in his establishment of the former Ludwig Boltzmann-Institute of Neurochemistry, in which pharmacological, biochemical and histopathological research into neuropsychiatric diseases was performed under one roof.

Further to his initial work on L-DOPA, Birkmayer has been in the forefront of supplementary parkinsonian therapy using enzyme inhibitors: benserazide in 1967, unselective monoamine oxidase inhibitors in 1962 and deprenyl in 1975.

Although theoretically in retirement, Birkmayer is more active than ever. As well as running two outpatient clinics, he has a large practice and regularly appears on Austrian television broadening popular understanding of neuropsychiatric problems. His research interests have not diminished either; he is continuing his search for better therapeutic strategies in Parkinson's disease and depression ("Die Parkinson-Krankheit"; Wien-New York: Springer 1980).

It has been twenty years ago since the neurochemical deficit in Parkinson's disease was identified. Where do we stand today? This volume, *dedicated to Prof. Dr. Walther Birkmayer on the occasion of his 70th anniversary*, attempts to answer that question, although there is little doubt that more questions than answers are forthcoming.

The Editors

Contents

Journal of Neural Transmission, Suppl. 16, 1—5 (1980)
© by Springer-Verlag 1980

Parkinson's Disease: Unanswered Questions

D. B. Calne and J. K. Kebabian

Experimental Therapeutics Branch, National Institute of Neurological and
Communicative Disorders and Stroke, Bethesda, Maryland, U.S.A.

Summary

Over the last two decades there have been spectacular advances in understanding and treating Parkinson's disease, but there remain major areas
of uncertainty and ignorance. The nigrostriatal pathway has features resembling the peripheral sympathetic system, rather than conventional central
projections of sensory and motor nuclei. Like sympathetic activity, nigrostriatal function is diffuse, tonic, and more accessible to analysis by
measuring biochemical rather than electrical changes. These findings are
difficult to interpret in the context of the established importance of the
basal ganglia in programming movement. The role of the depletion of
dopamine in Parkinsonism is also unclear; we do not even know whether
the impact of the deficit is more significant in the basal ganglia, or the
substantia nigra. Confusion over the actions of dopamine underlies the
obscurity of the mechanisms by which levodopa produces both wanted and
unwanted effects. Finally, the nature of Parkinson's disease is still an enigma:
we have not identified its cause, and we do not know what influences its
progress.

In attempting to elucidate the role of dopamine in brain function,
Parkinson's disease can be regarded as an experimental model
wrought by nature. The introduction of levodopa as treatment, a
development in which Prof. Birkmayer played such a pioneering
role, has been the most important therapeutic advance in neurology
over the last 20 years. But to avoid complacency, it is salutary
to consider the extent of our ignorance of related neuropharmacology. This exercise leads to such an extensive list of unanswered
problems that one may question whether the dimensions of a
scientific advance can be measured by the number of new questions
that it generates.

While the causal relationship between the dopamine deficit and the clinical syndrome is beyond doubt, the detailed analysis of the relationship is difficult, and no simple answers have been forthcoming. Under these circumstances it is timely to review our understanding and ignorance of the role of dopamine in the extrapyramidal nervous system and the etiology, pathology and prognosis of Parkinson's disease.

The Role of Dopamine

The major developments in our understanding of Parkinson's disease are the findings that (1) dopamine is depleted in the brain and (2) clinical improvement may be achieved with dopaminergic drugs. However, attempts to place these observations into a coherent framework of knowledge have been frustrated by the complexity of the task. If we wish to ascertain how a reduction of dopamine leads to rigidity, akinesia and tremor, it is reasonable to start by asking where, in terms of neuroanatomy, the depletion has a critical impact on function. This apparently simple question is not yet answerable. Framing the question more precisely, we cannot even state whether the crucial deficit for producing symptoms is in the nigra, the striatum, both, or neither. Drugs which deplete dopamine or block dopamine receptors are known to cause parkinsonism, but the category of receptors, and their location, remain obscure.

The anatomy, physiology and biochemistry of the dopaminergic nigroneostriatal projection displays features similar to the postganglionic sympathetic nervous system rather than the classical sensory or motor pathways in the mammalian nervous system. The sensorimotor systems have been amenable to intensive experimental investigation by single unit recording, because the spatial and temporal relationships between the peripheral events and the central electrical indicators of nervous activity are preserved with a high degree of fidelity. In a classical sensory or motor nucleus, excitatory and inhibitory synaptic input from presynaptic nerve terminals are integrated on the dendrites and soma of the postsynaptic neuron, whose axon becomes the final common pathway down which self-regenerating electrical discharges flow. At each relay station information is transmitted "point to point" with such precision that the peripheral sensory space, or pattern of muscle activation, can be mapped out within the nucleus.

The eye affords an example of an organ in which the differences between the sensorimotor and sympathetic nervous system are highlighted. The retina exemplifies a neural tissue in which the sensory information in encoded by the rate of discharge of neurons. This tissue displays an elaborate organization in which size, shape, location and movement of an image in the visual field is encoded by the rate of electrical discharge of neurons in a circumscribed region of the retina. Conversely, the iris provides an example of a tissue in which the time course of a response is considerably slower and in which there is little or no spatial organization. Furthermore, the crucial role of the sympathetic innervation of the dilator pupillae in regulating the amount of light which reaches the retina does not emerge from single unit analysis of the responses of the neurons within the retina.

Many of the features characteristic of the sympathetic nervous system can be identified in the nigroneostriatal dopaminergic neurons. First, these neurons display a slow tonic rate of electrical discharge. The combined biochemical and electrophysiological analysis of the discharge pattern of these dopaminergic neurons by Aghajanian and his coworkers has shown that drug treatments which cause massive biochemical changes are accompanied by only modest changes in the electrical responses of the dopaminergic neurons. The dopaminergic axons which project to the caudate nucleus arborize into a massive network reminiscent of the sympathetic innervation of peripheral effector organs. Within the rat brain, each caudate nucleus, weighing some 30 mg, receives its entire dopaminergic innervation from some 3500 cells whose soma reside in the substantia nigra. The combination of slow responses with anatomical divergence suggests that the dopaminergic neurons are not involved in "point to point" communications but are rather controlling more general (and as yet unidentified) physiological events in the caudate nucleus. In the case of the dopaminergic innervation of the striatum, it seems easier to look for chemical rather than electrical signs of nervous activity; this constitutes another analogy with the sympathetic system.

Recent neurochemical observations have raised the possibility that the axons of the dopaminergic neurons may not be the only "final common pathway" through which these cells influence activity in other neurons. Experimental evidence implies that the dendrites of the dopaminergic neurons may function as information-giving "presynaptic" elements. The demonstration of dopaminesensitive adenylate cyclase activity within the zona reticulata of the substantia nigra provides a receptor mechanism for dopamine; this enzyme activity is distinct from autoreceptors and is not associated with the dopaminergic neurons. The dendrites of the dopaminergic neurons are the only source of dopamine to interact with the cyclase receptor mechanisms, so presumably they establish dendrodentritic, dendrosomatic or dendro-axonal junctions between the zona compacta and in the zona reticulata of the substantia nigra. Thus, in any evaluation of the sites of action of dopamine within the extrapyramidal nervous system, it is necessary to consider the possibility that important events may occur outside the basal ganglia, in the substantia nigra.

Etiology, Pathology, Prognosis

Perhaps the most urgent unanswered question relating to Parkinson's disease concerns etiology. In spite of major advances in our analysis of the biochemical disturbances and the application of rational therapy, we still have no significant clues to the cause of the disorder. Current fashion attributes several neurological diseases of hitherto unknown origin to infection by an unconventional virus, or an abnormal immunological response to a conventional virus. There is no good evidence to implicate either of these mechanisms in the etiology of Parkinson's disease. Because Parkinson's disease is much commoner in the elderly, and some of its features have been construed as manifestations of senescence, there has been speculation that the disorder arises from accelerated or premature ageing of the central nervous system. However, the concept of ageing in this context is ill defined, so this hypothesis remains both unclear and unproven. The finding that infective, metabolic and toxic factors can induce a parkinsonian syndrome has proved unhelpful in the quest to explain the origin of the idiopathic disease.

The pathology of Parkinson's disease is another enigma. While degeneration of the nigrostriatal projection is usually found, *Denny Brown* has pointed out the paradox that the substantia nigra may occasionally appear normal in Parkinson's disease, and, furthermore, not all patients with lesions of the substantia nigra seem to develop the clinical features for Parkinsonism.

Since we do not know its etiology, and we are unsure of its pathology, it is not surprising that we are insecure in formulating a prognosis. The disease progresses at diverse rates in different individuals, and even within the same patient the speed of advance may alter. While the range, mean and variance of life expectation has been determined, we cannot predict the future for an individual with any precision, and we are unable to identify with any confidence those factors which are likely to increase or decrease the progress of the underlying neuropathology. There is even controversy over whether dopaminergic therapy should be started early or late in the course of the disease.

Adverse Reactions to Dopaminergic Agents

Since it is not yet possible to define the mechanism by which dopaminergic drugs achieve their therapeutic effect, it is not surprising that we do not understand how adverse reactions arise. Yet the latter problem is of the utmost practical importance in attempting to improve treatment, for an analysis of how unwanted effects develop should enable drugs to be designed with a higher therapeutic index. The major dose limiting adverse reactions to dopaminergic agents are dyskinesia, psychosis, and "on-off" reactions. We do not known the mechanism underlying any one of those problems, and we do not even have *in vitro* or *in vivo* analogues to facilitate screening new potentially therapeutic compounds. For example, in rodents dopaminergic drugs increase locomotor activity, cause stereotyped behavior, and induce turning in animals with unilateral nigral lesions. We cannot predict which, if any, of these effects might correlate with dyskinesia, psychosis, or a propensity for generating "on-off" reactions. Similarly, dopaminergic agents modify the concentration of other transmitters in the brain, but again we cannot state which of such changes might be useful and which deleterious. Since there are extremely high concentrations of so many neurotransmitters and neuromodulators in the nigrostriatal system, including acetylcholine and the peptides leu-enkephalin, met-enkephalin and substance P, it is tempting to speculate that a complex pattern of interacting and interdependent neurochemical activity is involved in motor function. But we cannot assign a role to all these agents—at present there are more actors than there are parts in the play!

Conclusion

Twenty years ago Prof. Birkmayer provided the clinical acumen and insight that elicited a therapeutic dividend from the advances in our understanding of the role of dopamine in the brain. Subsequent developments have led to the formulation of a plethora of new questions, and a deeper awareness of many persisting old questions.

Authors' address: *D. B. Calne*, D.M., F.R.C.P., Clinical Director, National Institute of Neurological and Communicative Disorders and Stroke, Building 10, Rm. 6D20, Bethesda, MD 20205, U.S.A.

Journal of Neural Transmission, Suppl. 16, 7—16 (1980)

Blood Platelets as Models for Neurons: Uses and Limitations

A. Pletscher and A. Laubscher

Department of Research, University Clinics, Basel, Switzerland

Summary

Platelets show similarities with 5-hydroxytryptaminergic neurons with respect to (1) uptake kinetics of 5-hydroxytryptamine (5-HT) at the plasma membrane, (2) inhibitory effects of tricyclic antidepressants and neuroleptics on 5-HT uptake, (3) granular storage of 5-HT and possibly catecholamines, (4) action of drugs interfering with granular and possibly extragranular amine storage and (5) reaction of the 5-HT receptor at the plasma membrane to 5-HT agonists and antagonists. Dissimilarities include (1) the uptake of catecholamines at the plasma membrane, (2) the biosynthesis of biogenic amines (absent in platelets, present in neurons) and (3) the turnover of 5-HT (slow or absent in platelets, fast in neurons). Although the above mentioned similarities are not absolute, platelets may be considered as reasonable models for some functions of 5-hydroxytryptaminergic neurons e.g. 5-HT uptake at the plasma membrane, intracellular storage of monoamines and reactions of 5-HT receptors to drugs. In addition, the shape change reaction of platelets can probably be used to identify those basic proteins and polypeptides which cause neuronal depolarization. The significance of disturbances of the monoamine system of platelets in neuropsychiatric disorders including Parkinson's syndrome is not yet clear in all respects. Therefore, some of the current ideas about the validity of platelets as models for neurons will be briefly reviewed in this article.

1. Amine Uptake

Various biogenic amines, e.g. 5-hydroxytryptamine (5-HT), dopamine (DA) and noradrenaline (NA), enter the platelets by passive diffusion. This uptake shows linear dependence on the external amine concentration and is not saturable. For 5-HT there exists a second uptake process, which has a high affinity for 5-HT (Table 1), is saturable and dependent on Na^+ and on metabolic energy. This carrier-mediated, specific uptake is much more efficient than the passive diffusion at low concentrations of the amine in the medium.

Table 1. *High affinity K_m values for uptake of monoamines and IC_{50} values of tricyclic drugs in isolated blood platelets and synaptosomes of guinea pigs at 37 °C*

			Synaptosomes	
Amine or drug		Platelets	Striatum	Hypothalamus
5-HT		$4.4 \pm 0.2 \times 10^{-7}$	$1.9 \pm 0.4 \times 10^{-7}$	$0.7 \pm 0.2 \times 10^{-7}$
DA	K_m^1 (M)	> 100	$1.3 \pm 0.3 \times 10^{-7}$	
NA		> 1000		$3.8 \pm 0.9 \times 10^{-7}$
Chlorimipramine		$1.1 \pm 0.3 \times 10^{-8}$	$5.2 \pm 1.5 \times 10^{-8}$	$2.5 \pm 0.7 \times 10^{-8}$
Imipramine		$2.6 \pm 0.3 \times 10^{-8}$	$3.2 \pm 0.8 \times 10^{-8}$	
Chlorpromazine	IC_{50}^2 (M)	$1.4 \pm 0.4 \times 10^{-7}$	$5.0 \pm 1.3 \times 10^{-7}$	$3.2 \pm 0.3 \times 10^{-7}$
Haloperidol		$1.1 \pm 0.1 \times 10^{-6}$	$2.6 \pm 0.7 \times 10^{-6}$	$2.0 \pm 0.5 \times 10^{-6}$

IC_{50} means concentration of the drugs in M causing 50 per cent inhibition of the uptake of 10^{-7} M ^3H-5-HT. Averages with S.E.M. of 4—7 experiments (*Pletscher et al.*, 1979).
[1] Platelets incubated in plasma.
[2] Platelets separated by a dextran gradient and incubated in Tris-buffer.

The specific uptake mechanism for 5-HT seems to be located at the plasma membrane. In fact, the initial 5-HT uptake measured in isolated plasma membranes of human platelets showed the same characteristics (K_m about 10^{-7} M, dependence on Na^+) and was inhibited by the same compounds (*e.g.* tricyclic antidepressants) as the 5-HT uptake in intact platelets (*Rudnick*, 1977). Also, in platelets in which the intracellular, granular storage of 5-HT was abolished by reserpine the K_m of the 5-HT uptake did not significantly differ from that in normal platelets (*e.g.* in guinea pigs 0.47 ± 0.06 versus 0.44 ± 0.02 μM, p > 0.05) (*Laubscher* and *Pletscher*, 1979).

The uptake of DA and NA in platelets is known to be much less pronounced than that of 5-HT. In guinea pigs, for instance it tended towards a saturation level only at very high concentrations of these amines, yielding an apparent K_m 2—3 orders higher than that of 5-HT (Table 1) (*Pletscher et al.*, 1979).

In neuronal tissue of the central nervous system (CNS), the uptake of 5-HT and of DA and NA at the plasma membrane has been shown to occur by a saturable, Na^+- and energy-dependent high affinity process. Thus, in guinea pigs the K_m values for the DA and NA uptake were 2—3 orders lower in neurons than in platelets (Table 1) indicating that platelets cannot be considered to provide a reasonable model for catecholaminergic neurons. On the other hand, the K_m values for 5-HT are of the same order in both neurons and platelets, although there may be differences between the two cell types in the affinities of the transport carriers for 5-HT.

2. Amine Storage

At the membrane of adrenal chromaffin granules there is probably a proton pump, driven by Mg^{++}-ATPase which creates an electrical and/or chemical gradient responsible for the catecholamine uptake. Evidence for such a mechanism also exists at the membrane of 5-HT granules (*Johnson et al.*, 1978). Once inside the granules, the amines probably form reversible aggregates with intragranular constituents such as ATP and proteins, thus being retained within the granules. The nature of these aggregates has been shown to be similar in 5-HT organelles of platelets and in catecholamine storage granules, *e.g.* of adrenal medulla, although certain differences may exist, for instance in the content of soluble proteins (*Pletscher,* 1978).

The granular storage of monoamines does not seem to show the same specificity as the uptake at the plasma membrane. In fact, in rabbits, the ratio of the amine concentrations in isolated 5-HT organelles to those in whole platelets were similar for 5-HT, DA, NA and adrenaline (259—376) whereas the absolute amount of 5-HT in whole platelets was more than 4 orders higher than that of the catecholamines (*Da Prada* and *Picotti,* 1979). In neuronal tissue, too, co-storage of various amines including false neurohumoral transmitters in the same organelles has been described (*Jaim-Etcheverry* and *Zieher,* 1975).

These and other findings indicate that the granular storage of biogenic monoamines in platelets is similar in many respects to that in neurons. Exact comparisons between the 5-HT storage organelles of platelets and those of 5-hydroxytryptaminergic neurons should, however, be made to confirm and supplement the current ideas on this subject.

Extragranular storage sites for monoamines seem to occur in neuronal cells. Experiments with drugs (see below) also point to the existence of such sites in platelets but these results remain to be substantiated.

3. Uptake Inhibition and Release

3.1. Site of Action

The sites of action of inhibitors of 5-HT uptake can be partly differentiated by comparing the effects of the inhibitors in normal and in reserpinized platelets, *i.e.* those in which the granular storage has been abolished.

Inhibitors whose principal site of action is the plasma membrane should show the same IC_{50} (concentration of the inhibitor causing half maximal inhibition of the uptake of 10^{-7} M 5-HT) in both normal and reserpinized platelets. This gives a quotient $IC_{50}R/IC_{50}N$ of about 1 (R = reserpinized, N = normal platelets). In contrast, the IC_{50} of inhibitors which act preferentially at the intracellular storage organelles should be much higher in reserpinized than in normal platelets, leading to a quotient $IC_{50}R/IC_{50}N$ considerably greater than 1. Indeed, tricyclic antidepressants and neuroleptics, which exert their inhibitory action preferentially at the plasma membrane, showed

Table 2. *Effect of inhibitors of 5-HT uptake in normal (N) and reserpinized (R) human platelets*

Substance	$IC_{50}N$	$IC_{50}R$	$IC_{50}R/IC_{50}N$
Imipramine	4.2 ± 0.2	4.6 ± 0.3	1.1 ± 0.0
Ro 4-1284	21.3 ± 1.4	$> 10^4$	> 100
Chlorimipramine	0.5 ± 0.1	0.5 ± 0.1	1.0 ± 1.1
Desmethylimipramine	52.0 ± 2.1	59.0 ± 1.5	1.1 ± 0.0
Amitryptiline	9.7 ± 1.2	11.1 ± 2.0	1.1 ± 0.1
Chlorpromazine	65.3 ± 10.6	66.3 ± 4.2	1.1 ± 0.2
Haloperidol	$15.1 \pm 1.6 \times 10^2$	$33.7 \pm 1.5 \times 10^2$	2.3 ± 0.3
Spiroperidol	$31.3 \pm 3.3 \times 10^2$	$78.3 \pm 8.0 \times 10^2$	2.5 ± 0.2
Prenylamine	$2.6 \pm 0.4 \times 10^2$	$15.7 \pm 1.7 \times 10^2$	6.5 ± 1.5
Ro 4-9040	51.2 ± 15.9	536.4 ± 119.1	11.5 ± 1.7
N', N'-Dimethyl-tryptamine	$14.0 \pm 1.1 \times 10^2$	$8.9 \pm 1.0 \times 10^2$	0.6 ± 0.0
p-Chlormet-amphetamine	$6.2 \pm 0.1 \times 10^2$	$4.8 \pm 0.5 \times 10^2$	0.8 ± 0.1

Platelet-rich plasma was preincubated with 2×10^{-6} M reserpine (final concentration) or solvent at 37 °C for 30 min. The platelets were then isolated on a dextran gradient and reincubated at 37 °C for 10 min in Tris-buffer with the drugs. Thereafter ^{3}H-5-HT (10^{-7} M final concentration) was added and the incubation continued for another 5 min. The incubation was stopped by adding 3 vol. of 2% formaldehyde and the radioactivity of the isolated platelets measured (*Laubscher* and *Pletscher*, 1979 a). IC_{50} values are indicated in nM. Averages with S.E.M. of 3—4 experiments.

a quotient of about 1. In contrast, the benzoquinolizine derivative Ro 4-1284, which has a relatively selective action on the 5-HT granules, had a quotient of more than 100. There were also drugs with a quotient between 1 and 100, *e.g.* haloperidol, Ro 4-9040 and prenylamine. They probably exert an effect on granular storage but in addition on the plasma membrane and/or on extragranular sites. Some compounds (*e.g.* N′, N′-dimethyltryptamine and p-chlormetamphetamine) had a quotient below 1, indicating that an effect on extragranular, intracellular sites is a component of their action (Table 2).

Comparisons of reserpinized with normal platelets may provide clues to the site of action of drugs in 5-hydroxytryptaminergic neurons since the uptake and storage mechanisms of 5-HT in platelets seem to be similar to those in neurons.

3.2. Plasma Membrane

In general, the drugs which preferentially interfere with the uptake of 5-HT at the plasma membrane are effective in both platelets and in neurons. Tricyclic antidepressants and neuroleptics have even been shown to have a similar order of potencies in platelets and synaptosomes (Table 1) (*Pletscher*, 1978). Whether such a close correlation also exists for other classes of drugs remains to be further clarified.

3.3. Granular Storage Sites

The granular storage of monoamines can be disturbed by agents leading to exocytosis and by reserpine- and tyramine-like drugs. In exocytosis the whole granular content (including nucleotides, soluble proteins etc.) is discarded. Reserpine- and tyramine-like drugs mainly affect the storage of the amines but they differ in their mechanisms: reserpine probably acts at the granular membrane level whereas tyramine displaces the intragranular amines from their storage complexes (*Pletscher*, 1978).

In monoaminergic neurons as well as in platelets granular amines can be released by exocytosis, although the physiological stimuli are probably not the same (*e.g.* electrical in neurons, thrombin in platelets). Furthermore, in both cell types numerous reserpine-like drugs inhibit granular amine uptake and amine release, and granular amines are also displaced by various phenyl- and indolylalkylamines (*Laubscher* and *Pletscher*, 1979). However, an exact comparison has not yet been made between the potencies of these drugs in interfering with the granular storage of 5-HT, DA and NA in neurons and in platelets.

3.4. Extragranular, Intracellular Sites

Tryptamine- and amphetamine-derivatives have been reported to inhibit 5-HT-accumulation more markedly in synaptosomes from reserpinized rats than in those from normal animals, probably due to interference of the drugs with the extragranular accumulation of 5-HT (*Ross*, 1979). Therefore, these drugs seem to act in a similar way in neurons as in platelets, in which they showed a quotient $IC_{50}R/IC_{50}N$ below 1 (Table 2).

4. The Platelet Shape Change

The shape change reaction of platelets is characterized by a transition from the normally occurring discoid shape into a spheroid form leading to an increase in the light absorption of the platelet suspensions. Under the conditions used in the following experiments, *i.e.* in artificial buffer systems, there is no platelet aggregation to interfere with the results (*Graf* and *Pletscher*, 1979).

4.1. The 5-HT Receptor

5-HT-induced a shape change reaction which was markedly inhibited by 5-HT antagonists such as methysergide and spiroperidol (Table 3). Among the various biogenic amines tested only tryptamine-

Table 3. *Potencies of various drugs as antagonists of 5-HT receptors in platelets and cerebral cortex*

	Potencies			
	Platelets		Cerebral cortex	
Compounds	Man[1]	Rabbit[1]	Monkey[2]	Rat[3]
Spiroperidol	$2.2 \pm 0.4 \times 10^{-9}$	$1.0 \pm 0.1 \times 10^{-9}$	8	8.5
Methiothepin	$4.1 \pm 0.2 \times 10^{-9}$	$1.2 \pm 0.1 \times 10^{-9}$	11	8.2
Cyproheptadine		$2.1 \pm 0.1 \times 10^{-9}$	29	
Methysergide	$1.4 \pm 0.1 \times 10^{-8}$	$6.2 \pm 0.7 \times 10^{-9}$	42	
Chlorpromazine	$2.8 \pm 0.5 \times 10^{-8}$	$6.8 \pm 0.6 \times 10^{-9}$	64	7.2
D-Butaclamol	$1.7 \pm 0.3 \times 10^{-8}$	$1.3 \pm 0.1 \times 10^{-8}$		7.0
Haloperidol	$3.4 \pm 0.0 \times 10^{-7}$	$1.8 \pm 0.4 \times 10^{-7}$	40	6.9
L-Butaclamol	$3.2 \pm 0.4 \times 10^{-6}$	$> 10^{-5}$		

[1] 5-HT-induced shape change: IC_{50} values in M (*Laubscher* and *Pletscher*, 1979 a).

[2] Antagonism against 5-HT-stimulated adenylate cyclase in anterior limbic cortex: K_i values (*Ahn* and *Makman*, 1978).

[3] Inhibition of ^3H-spiroperidol binding in frontal cortex: $-\log IC_{50}$ (*Leysen et al.*, 1978).

derivatives (but not precursors or metabolites) and other substances known to be 5-HT agonists caused a shape change reaction. Some compounds were mixed agonists–antagonists (Table 4). There was also a marked stereoselectivity since D-LSD and D-butaclamol showed potencies several orders higher than their corresponding L-isomers. These findings strongly indicate that the 5-HT-induced shape change reaction is mediated by the stimulation of a specific 5-HT receptor.

Table 4. *EC_{50} (molar concentration of drug causing half maximal shape change) and IC_{50} (molar concentration of drug causing 50 % inhibition of shape change due to 10^{-6} M 5-HT) of 5-HT agonists and mixed 5-HT agonists–antagonists in human platelets incubated in citrate buffer*

Drug	Agonist EC_{50}	Antagonist IC_{50}
5-HT	$1.4 \pm 0.1 \times 10^{-7}$	
D-LSD	$9.9 \pm 1.2 \times 10^{-9}$	$4.3 \pm 0.4 \times 10^{-9}$
N', N'-Dimethyl-5-HT*	$1.3 \pm 0.4 \times 10^{-7}$	$4.5 \pm 0.4 \times 10^{-7}$
Tryptamine	$1.4 \pm 0.3 \times 10^{-6}$	
N', N'-Dimethyltryptamine	$2.0 \pm 0.9 \times 10^{-6}$	$2.0 \pm 1.1 \times 10^{-6}$
Quipazine*	$2.0 \pm 0.4 \times 10^{-6}$	
Mescaline	$2.0 \pm 0.5 \times 10^{-5}$	
L-LSD	$> 10^{-5}$	$1.9 \pm 0.3 \times 10^{-5}$

Averages with S.E.M. of 3—4 experiments (*Laubscher* and *Pletscher*, 1979 a; *Graf* and *Pletscher*, 1979).

* Rabbit platelets.

The same compounds seem to act as 5-HT agonists in the CNS and in platelets *e.g.* tryptamine- and 5-HT-derivatives, quipazine and mescaline. For 5-HT antagonists there are some discrepancies between platelets and neurons, possibly due to the existence of various types of 5-HT receptors in the CNS. In areas with a dense 5-hydroxy-tryptaminergic innervation (raphé nuclei, amygdala, ventral lateral, geniculate, optic tectum) various compounds have been reported to act as 5-HT agonists which were potent 5-HT antagonists in platelets. In the hippocampus, too, the neuronal 5-HT receptors were not exactly comparable to those of platelets in their reaction to antag-onists. However, in other regions of the CNS (*e.g.* spinal cord, cortex) platelets and neurons reacted similarly (*Pletscher et al.*, 1979; *Graf* and *Pletscher*, 1979). For instance, the orders of potencies of various neuroleptic drugs and other 5-HT antagonists were reasonably parallel in both cell types (Table 3) (*Laubscher* and *Pletscher*, 1979 a).

Therefore, the 5-HT receptors of platelets seem to react to the same 5-HT agonists and antagonists as the neuronal 5-HT receptors of some areas of the CNS.

4.2. Basic Proteins

Basic proteins and polypeptides (BPP) such as myelin basic protein (MBP), polyornithine, polylysine and protamine also caused a marked shape change reaction in platelets suspended in artificial medium. This shape change was not due to stimulation of 5-HT or other receptors since it could not be counteracted by antagonists of 5-HT (methysergide and spiroperidol), DA, NA and GABA. The BPP are positively charged and by attaching themselves to the negatively charged plasma membrane of the platelets may trigger off the shape change reaction. The finding that the acid mucopolysaccharide heparin antagonized the shape change caused by BPP lends support to this view (*Laubscher et al.*, 1979).

It is of interest that the shape change-inducing action of BPP depends on their molecular weight and conformation. For instance, low molecular weight polyornithine (M.W. 4000) and cytochrome C, a basic non-random coil protein did not cause a shape change reaction in contrast to the higher molecular weight polyornithine (M.W. 40,000). The polyamines spermine and spermidine were also inactive.

It has been reported that neuronal cells are affected by the same BPP as platelets. In fact, MBP, polyornithine 40,000, polylysine and protamine inhibited the electrical activity of neurons in the spinal cord *in situ* and/or of cultured neuronal cells *in vitro*. Antagonists of DA, NA and GABA did not counteract these effects. Other basic substances *e.g.* spermine, spermidine, cytochrome C and polyornithine 4000 were inactive (*Honegger et al.*, 1977; *Gähwiler* and *Honegger*, 1979).

From these findings it may be concluded that the shape change reaction of platelets is a sensitive and simple means of detecting those BPP which cause functional changes in neuronal cells. Platelets could also be used as models to screen for substances inhibiting the membrane effects of BPP. This is of interest because of the speculation that some neurological manifestations in the course of demyelinating disorders such as multiple sclerosis (*Gähwiler* and *Honegger*, 1979), or in cerebral stroke, are due to a direct action of MBP on neuronal membranes.

References

Ahn, H. S., Makman, M. H.: Serotonin sensitive adenylate cyclase activity in monkey anterior limbic cortex: Antagonism by molindone and other antipsychotic drugs. Life Sci. *23*, 507—511 (1978).

Da Prada, M., Picotti, G. B.: Content and subcellular localization of catecholamines and 5-hydroxytryptamine in human and animal blood platelets: Monoamine distribution between platelets and plasma. Brit. J. Pharmac. *65*, 653—662 (1979).

Gähwiler, B. H., Honegger, C. G.: Myelin basic protein depolarizes neuronal membranes. Neurosci. Lett. *11*, 317—321 (1979).

Graf, M., Pletscher, A.: Shape change of blood platelets—a model for cerebral 5-hydroxytryptamine receptors? Br. J. Pharmac. *65*, 601—608 (1979).

Honegger, C. G., Gähwiler, B. H., Isler, H.: The effect of myelin basic protein (MBP) on the bioelectric activity of spinal cord and cerebellar neurons. Neurosci. Lett. *4*, 303—307 (1977).

Jaim-Etcheverry, G., Zieher, L. M.: Octopamine probably coexists with noradrenaline and serotonin in vesicles of pineal adrenergic nerves. J. Neurochem. *25*, 915—917 (1975).

Johnson, R. G., Scarpa, A., Salganicoff, L.: The internal pH of isolated serotonin containing granules of pig platelets. J. Biol. Chem. *253*, 7061—7068 (1978).

Laubscher, A., Pletscher, A.: Uptake of 5-hydroxytryptamine in blood platelets and its inhibition by drugs: role of plasma membrane and granular storage. J. Pharm. Pharmacol. *31*, 284—289 (1979).

Laubscher, A., Pletscher, A.: Shape change and uptake of 5-hydroxytryptamine in human blood platelets: Action of neuropsychotropic drugs. Life Sci. *24*, 1833—1840 (1979 a).

Laubscher, A., Pletscher, A., Honegger, C. G., Richards, J. G., Colombo, V.: Shape change of blood platelets induced by myelin basic protein. Experientia *35*, 1081—1082 (1979).

Leysen, J. E., Niemegeers, C. J. E., Tollenaere, J. P., Laduron, P. M.: Serotonergic component of neuroleptic receptors. Nature *272*, 168—171 (1978).

Pletscher, A.: Platelets as models for monoaminergic neurons. In: Essays in Neurochemistry and Neuropharmacology, Vol. 3, p. 49. London: John Wiley and Sons Ltd. 1978.

Pletscher, A., Laubscher, A., Graf, M., Saner, A.: Blood platelets as models for central 5-hydroxytryptaminergic neurons. Ann. Biol. Clin. *37*, 35—39 (1979).

Ross, S. B.: Interactions between reserpine and various compounds on the accumulation of [^{14}C]5-hydroxytryptamine and [^{3}H]noradrenaline in homogenates from rat hypothalamus. Biochem. Pharmacol. *28*, 1085—1088 (1979).

Rudnick, G.: Active transport of 5-hydroxytryptamine by plasma membrane vesicles isolated from human blood platelets. J. Biol. Chem. *252,* 2170—2174 (1977).

Authors' address: Prof. Dr. *A. Pletscher,* Department of Research, Kantons-spital Basel, Hebelstrasse 20, CH-4031 Basel, Switzerland.

Journal of Neural Transmission, Suppl. 16, 17—23 (1980)
© by Springer-Verlag 1980

Changing Concepts of Nigral Dopamine System Function Within the Basal Ganglia: Relevance to Extrapyramidal Disorders*

B. S. Bunney, A. A. Grace, and D. W. Hommer

Departments of Psychiatry and Pharmacology, Yale University School of Medicine,
New Haven, Connecticut, U.S.A.

Summary

The recent discovery of new methods for tracing brain pathways and studying their function has greatly expanded our knowledge of the areas of the brain involved in extrapyramidal disorders and has begun to change our concept of how these areas function. One such change has involved our understanding of the role of the dopaminergic system within the basal ganglia. Rather than dopamine being seen primarily as a major influence on striatal output it is now perhaps best conceptualized as one link in a set of circular pathways, one of whose functions is to modulate non-dopaminergic output from the substantia nigra to other brain regions. In addition, new evidence suggests that this neurotransmitter system may play a role in the way sensory inputs are handled by the basal ganglia. These new roles for the nigral dopaminergic system raise important new questions about its function in extrapyramidal motor systems as well as provide possible answers to questions concerning the mechanisms underlying some of the symptoms seen in disorders involving the basal ganglia.

Accidental discoveries have been responsible for most of the breakthroughs in the pharmacological treatment of CNS diseases. The development of L-dopa treatment in Parkinson's disease (*Birkmayer* and *Hornykiewicz*, 1961, 1962) stands out as the rare exception in which a knowledge of the pathology underlying the disease led to a rational choice of therapy. The fact that serendipitous observations have been the primary method for significant pharmacological discoveries until recently, is not surprising given the

* This work was supported by NIH Grants # 28849, # 25642 and GM-07527.

enormous complexity of the brain and the relatively little that we know about its architecture and function. However, the recent development of numerous new methodologies and sophisticated research instrumentation has provided the investigator with a powerful new armamentarium of approaches for studying the central nervous system. Perhaps nowhere in the brain have the new methodologies been used more extensively to expand our knowledge than in studies of the areas believed to be involved in the pathogenesis of Parkinson's disease, Huntington's chorea and the neurological side effects of antipsychotic drugs—the so-called extrapyramidal system. It is beyond the scope of this chapter to review all of the new anatomical, behavioral, biochemical and electrophysiological discoveries that have been made concerning this system. Therefore, we have arbitrarily chosen a few to discuss which, from our point of view, appear important. Possible new roles of the dopaminergic (DA) system within the basal ganglia and their relevance to extrapyramidal disorders will be our main consideration.

It used to be thought that only about 5 % of all the neurons in the caudate nucleus were output neurons and that most efferents from the caudate nucleus travelled only as far as the globus pallidus where they made synaptic contact with cells which then proceeded to the thalamus and thence to the cortex (*Kemp* and *Powell,* 1971). However, recent studies using a variety of techniques, including retrograde tracing with horseradish peroxidase and autoradiography, have suggested that as many as 50 % of the cells in the caudate nucleus (in the cat and rat) project to the substantia nigra (*Grofova,* 1975; *Bunney* and *Aghajanian,* 1976). Such studies also have demonstrated that there are neurons in the globus pallidus which project back to the substantia nigra (*Hattori et al.,* 1975). Two neurotransmitters used by links in these pathways appear to be GABA (*McGeer et al.,* 1974) and substance P (*Hong et al.,* 1977). Until very recently it had been hypothesized that the major role of these so-called feedback pathways from the striatum to the substantia nigra was the modulation of DA cell activity and consequently regulation of the influence of the nigral DA system on the caudate nucleus and its projections via the globus pallidus to the thalamus. However, recent behavioral and electrophysiological studies suggest that in addition to modulating DA cell activity the projections from the striatum to the substantia nigra may form a major output system of the striatum to the thalamus and other parts of the brain (*Garcia-Munoz et al.,* 1977; *York* and *Faber,* 1977; *Arnt* and *Scheel-Krüger,* 1979; *DiChiara et al.,* 1979). Of particular interest are anatomical studies which have demonstrated projections from the substantia nigra to the thalamus and the superior colliculus (*Clavier et al.*, 1976; *Graybiel*, 1978; *Bentivoglio et al.*, 1979). The latter pathway appears to be GABA-ergic and may be inhibitory (*Vincent et al.*, 1978).

Recently, we have found that within the zona reticulata there is a non-DA neuron which is approximately 20 times more sensitive to the inhibition induced by iontophoretically administered GABA than is the DA neuron itself (*Grace* and *Bunney*, 1979). This neuron appears to exert an inhibitory influence upon DA cells which is blocked by the GABA antagonist picrotoxin, suggesting that the zona reticulata neuron might use GABA as its neurotransmitter. Since the zona reticulata neuron is many times more sensitive to the inhibitory effects of GABA than is the DA cell, one might expect that locally and/or systemically administered muscimol would have a preferential effect on zona reticulata cells. Thus, the zona reticulata cell would be inhibited and the DA cell disinhibited. Measurement of dopamine metabolites in the caudate nucleus after local administration of muscimol into the substantia nigra suggests that DA cells are indeed activated (*Biggio et al.*, 1977; *Waddington*, 1977). In addition, several investigators have shown that intravenous muscimol induces an increase in the activity of DA neurons (*Walters* and *Lakoski*, 1978; *McNeil et al.*, 1978; *Grace* and *Bunney*, 1979).

The question arises as to whether or not this GABA sensitive neuron in the zona reticulata is an interneuron or an output neuron with collaterals to DA cells. Neurons in the zona reticulata can be activated antidromically by stimulation in the thalamus and superior colliculus (*Anderson* and *Yoshida*, 1977). In preliminary studies, we have confirmed this observation and demonstrated that stimulation in the ventral medial nucleus of the thalamus or the intermediate gray of the superior colliculus induces an inhibition of DA neurons whose magnitude of inhibition is significantly decreased by intravenous picrotoxin (*Grace* and *Bunney*, in preparation).

Thus, GABA-ergic striatonigral pathways may preferentially inhibit non-DA nigral zona reticulata neurons (which may be themselves GABA-ergic) some of which project to the superior colliculus and/or thalamus while at the same time sending collaterals to the zona compacta DA neurons.

Exactly what the consequences of the existence of such a circuit are for behavior is not yet clear. However, one can speculate that malfunctions within the system may be responsible for some of the symptoms one sees in a variety of extrapyramidal disorders. Thus, abnormalities of eye movement are found in patients suffering from Huntington's Chorea (*Avanzini et al.*, 1979) and Parkinson's disease (*Jones* and *DeJong*, 1971). The abnormalities involve horizontal and vertical saccadic eye movements. As the superior colliculus is known to be involved in such movements (*Wurtz* and *Goldberg*, 1972) the nigrotectal pathway, which is under DA and GABA-ergic influences, would provide one possible anatomical connection for the mediation of these symptoms. Based on their data *Wurtz* and *Goldberg* (1972) hypothesized that the superior colliculus may be involved in *initiation* of eye movement and the shifting of attention from one visual stimulus to the next. It may be more than a coincidence that the striatum and pallidum, with which the superior colliculus now appears to be connected (indirectly), is also thought to be involved in initiation of movement (*DeLong*, 1971).

The existence of a nigrotectal system which is influenced by a DA-system through striatal efferents may also explain some of the side effects of antipsychotic drugs. For example, a small percentage of patients treated with antipsychotic drugs (especially adolescents) develop an acute dystonic reaction which may include oculogyric crisis (*Klein* and *Davis*, 1969). Disturbance of the superior colliculus can lead to abnormalities of upward gaze (*Apter*, 1945). Acute blockade of dopamine receptors on neurons forming part of the striatonigral feedback pathway or of DA autoreceptors could affect, indirectly, the functioning of this nucleus through the circuits described above. The fact that a variety of drugs are effective in treating this disorder may be explained by hypothesizing that intervention at any of a number of points along the pathways which mediate upward gaze will restore whatever imbalance has been induced by the antipsychotic drug.

Another example of new discoveries which are changing the way we view the role of the DA system within the basal ganglia is the finding that the activity of nigrostriatal DA neurons can be affected by external stimuli. The first clues that this might be the case came from the biochemical work of *Nieoullon et al.* (1977). Subsequently, light flashes and tail pressure were found to activate DA neurons (*Chiodo et al.*, 1979). In preliminary experiments we (*Hommer* and *Bunney*, in preparation) have found that brief electrical stimulation of the sciatic nerve or noxious pressure applied to the tail or foot causes a transient depression of DA cell activity often followed by a series of subsequent oscillations between excitation and inhibition with a subsequent rapid return to baseline firing rate. These oscillations can be blocked by administering low doses of haloperidol (0.1 mg/kg i.v.) suggesting that DA receptors (perhaps on striatonigral feedback pathway neurons) are somehow involved in the mechanism responsible for the oscillations. The initial stimulus-induced inhibition of the DA neurons is blocked by low doses of picrotoxin (1 mg/kg) suggesting that a GABA-ergic neuron is involved somewhere in the input circuit. For example, a population of non-DA zona reticulata neurons have been found that appear to have an exact reciprocal activity relationship with the DA cells (*Grace* and *Bunney,* 1979) and have a nearly identical latency of response to sciatic nerve stimulation (*Hommer* and *Bunney,* in preparation). These cells are extremely sensitive to inhibition by GABA and appear to be the same ones which inhibit DA cells, an effect which is blocked by low doses of picrotoxin. The identification of these cells as belonging to the nigrothalamic or nigrotectal system has yet to be carried out.

These findings would suggest that incoming external stimuli can set up oscillations in the activity of zona compacta DA neurons (perhaps through an input to the GABA sensitive non-DA zona reticulata neurons) which under normal conditions are rapidly damped away. Is it possible that such damping may *not* occur in disease states involving the basal ganglia (*e.g.* Huntington's chorea) and therefore lead to prolonged marked and rapid oscillations in the activity of the nigrostriatal DA system?

In summary, the development of new methodological techniques has been responsible for the rapid advance in our knowledge of the anatomy and functioning of the basal ganglia and thus a corresponding advancement in our understanding of the pathogenesis of basal ganglia disorders. It now seems only a matter of time before our knowledge will expand to the point that rational new pharmacological therapies for these disorders can be developed. For example, because it is known that Parkinson patients suffer from a deficiency of dopamine in the brain most of our therapeutic approaches to the treatment of that disorder are devoted to replacing the dopamine in one form or another (*i.e.* either through the administration of a precursor or other drugs which stimulate dopamine receptors directly). However, as we know more about the circuitry of the basal ganglia and the neurotransmitters used by that circuitry it should be possible to design new drugs for the treatment of Parkinsonism which act on systems "downstream" from the destroyed DA system and thereby provide rational new approaches to the treatment of Parkinson's disease.

In addition, as we learn more about the basal ganglia our conception of the role that the DA system plays within it is changing. Already it is becoming evident that, rather than its major function being modulation of caudate nucleus cell output, the nigral DA system may be a link in a circular circuit, whose functions may include modulation of sensory input to the basal ganglia as well as output from the substantia nigra.

References

Anderson, M., Yoshida, M.: Electrophysiological evidence for branching nigral projections to the thalamus and the superior colliculus. Brain Res. *137,* 361—364 (1977).

Apter, J. T.: Eye movements following strychninzation of the superior colliculus of cats. J. Neurophysiol. *9,* 73—86 (1946).

Arnt, J., Scheel-Krüger, J.: GABA-ergic and glycinergic mechanisms within the substantia nigra: Pharmacological specificity of dopamine-independent contralateral turning behavior and interactions with other neurotransmitters. Psychopharmacol. *62,* 267—277 (1979).

Avanzini, G., Girotti, F., Caraceni, T., Spreafico, R.: Oculomotor disorders in Huntington's chorea. J. Neurol. Neurosurg. Psychiat. *42,* 581—589 (1979).

Bentivoglio, M., Van Derkooy, D., Kuypers, H. G. J. M.: The organization of the efferent projections of the substantia nigra in the rat. A retrograde fluorescent double labeling study. Brain Res. *174,* 1—7 (1979).

Biggio, G., Caso, M., Corda, M. G., Vernaleone, F., Gessa, G. L.: Effect of muscimol, a GABA-mimetic agent, on dopamine metabolism in the mouse brain. Life Sci. *21,* 525—532 (1977).

Birkmayer, W., Hornykiewicz, O.: Der L-Dioxyphenylalanin (= L-Dopa)- Effekt bei der Parkinson-Akinese. Wien. klin. Wschr. *73,* 787 (1961).

Birkmayer, W., Hornykiewicz, O.: Der L-Dioxyphenylalanin (= L-Dopa)- Effekt beim Parkinson-Syndrom des Menschen. Zur Pathogenese und Behandlung der Parkinson-Akinese. Arch. Psychiat. Nervenkr. *203,* 560—574 (1962).

Bunney, B. S., Aghajanian, G. K.: The precise localization of nigral afferents in the rat as determined by a retrograde tracing technique. Brain Res. *117,* 423—435 (1976).

Chiodo, L. A., Caggiula, A. R., Antelman, S. M., Lineberry, C. G.: Reciprocal influences of activating and immobilizing stimuli on the activity of nigrostriatal dopamine neurons. Brain Res. 1979 (in press).

Clavier, R. M., Atmodja, S., Fibiger, H. C.: Nigrothalamic projections in the rat as demonstrated by orthograde and retrograde tracing techniques. Brain Res. Bull. *1,* 379—384 (1976).

DeLong, M. R.: Activity of pallidal neurons during movement. J. Neurophysiol. *34,* 414—427 (1971).

DiChiara, G., Porceddu, M. L., Morelli, M., Mulas, M. L., Gessa, G. L.: Substantia nigra as an out-put station for striatal dopaminergic responses: Role of GABA-mediated inhibition of pars reticulata neurons. Naunyn-Schmiedeberg's Arch. Pharmacol. *306,* 153—159 (1979).

Grace, A., Bunney, B. S.: GABA agonist excitation of nigral dopamine cells: Mediation through reticulata inhibitory neurons. Europ. J. Pharmacol. (1979) in press.

Graybiel, A. M.: The organization of the nigrotectal connection: An experimental tracer study in the cat. Brain Res. *143,* 339—348 (1978).

Grofova, I.: The identification of striatal and pallidal neurons projecting to substantia nigra. An experimental study by means of retrograde axonal transport of horseradish peroxidase. Brain Res. *91,* 286—291 (1975).

Hattori, T., Fibiger, H. C., McGeer, P. L.: Demonstration of a pallido-nigral projection innervating dopaminergic neurons. J. Comp. Neur. *162,* 487—504 (1975).

Hong, J. S., Yang, H.-Y. T., Racagni, G., Costa, E.: Projections of substance P containing neurons from neostriatum to substantia nigra. Brain Res. *122,* 541—544 (1977).

Jones, G. M., DeJong, J. D.: Dynamic characteristics of saccadic eye movements in Parkinson's disease. Exp. Neurol. *31,* 17—31 (1971).

Kemp, J. M., Powell, T. P. S.: The structure of the caudate nucleus of the cat: Light and electron microscopy. Phil. Trans. R. Soc. Lond. *262,* 383—401 (1971).

Klein, D. E., Davis, J. M.: Diagnosis and Drug Treatment of Psychiatric Disorders, p. 95. Baltimore: The Williams and Wilkins Company. 1969.

Mac Neil, D., Ganer, M., Szymanska, I.: Response of dopamine neurons in substantia nigra to muscimol. Brain Res. *154,* 401—403 (1978).

McGeer, P. L., Fibiger, H. C., Hattori, T., Singh, V. K., McGeer, E. G., Maler, L.: Biochemical neuroanatomy of the basal ganglia. In: Advances in Behavioral Biology, Vol. 10 (*Myers, R. D., Drucker-Colin, R. R.,* eds.), pp. 27—47. New York: Plenum Press. 1974.

Nieoullon, A., Cheramy, A., Glowinski, J.: Nigral and striatal dopamine release under sensory stimuli. Nature *269,* 340—342 (1977).

Vincent, S. R., Hattori, T., McGeer, E. G.: The nigrotectal projection: A biochemical and ultrastructural characterization. Brain Res. *151,* 159 to 164 (1978).

Waddington, J. C.: GABA-like properties of flurazepam and baclofen suggested by rotational behavior following unilateral intranigral injection: A comparison with the GABA agonist muscimol. Br. J. Pharmacol. *60,* 263P—264P (1977).

Walters, J. R., Lakoski, J. M.: Effect of muscimol on single unit activity of substantia nigra dopamine neurons. Europ. J. Pharmacol. *47,* 469—471 (1978).

York, D. H., Faber, J. E.: An electrophysiological study of nigrotectal relationships: A possible role in turning behavior. Brain Res. *130,* 383—386 (1977).

Authors' address: *B. S. Bunney,* M.D., Neuropsychopharmacology Research Unit, Yale University School of Medicine, 333 Cedar Street, New Haven, CT 06510, U.S.A.

Journal of Neural Transmission, Suppl. 16, 25—31 (1980)
© by Springer-Verlag 1980

An Autoradiographic Study of the Striatofugal Fibers in the Monkey*

L. J. Poirier** and **Monique Giguère**

Laboratoire de Neurobiologie and Département de Médecine, Université Laval, and Hôpital de l'Enfant-Jésus, Québec, Canada

With 10 Figures

Summary

Anterograde labelling with ^{3}H-leucine was used to study the course and termination of striatofugal fibers in the monkey. Following injection of the isotope in the most medial part of the head and the body of the caudate nucleus fibers were traced along the ventrolateral part of the internal capsule and within the medial part of the comb bundle before penetrating the rostromedial pole of the substantia nigra (SN). Fiber endings were found along the dorsomedial edge of both divisions of the pallidum and in approximately the medial third of the SN over the whole length of this structure. Injection in the rostromedial part of the putamen resulted in silver grain concentrations representing labelled terminals in the central part of both divisions of the pallidum and in the ventrolateral and central part of the SN. Isotope concentration was equally important in both parts, reticulata and compacta, of the SN. These results favour the existence of rostrocaudal and mediolateral topographical relationships between, on the one end, the neostriatum and, on the other end, the pallidum and the SN.

The origin, course and termination of the striatofugal fibers were studied in two monkeys. The isotope (^{3}H-leucine) (30 μCi of a solution of 3.0 μl) was slowly injected into the caudate nucleus and putamen using a Hamilton 1 μl syringue fitted with a 31 gauge needle. The procedure of *Cowan et al.* (1977) was followed for the prepara-

---

* Supported by the Medical Research Council of Canada.
** Holder of a Killam Memorial Scholarship.

tion of the brains and the demonstration of the radioactive material on sections of the nervous tissue. The animals were allowed to survive 5 and 6 days following the injection of the radioactive amino acid. Serial sections were mounted, coated with Kodak NTB2 emulsion and exposed at 4 °C for 10 days to 9 weeks. Then they were developed in D-170 (local formula) and stained with a basic dye.

In two monkeys (1 macaque and 1 squirrel) the injection of the isotope heavily labelled the most medial part of the right caudate nucleus (Fig. 1) over approximately the rostral two thirds of this structure. In the macaque H³-leucine was also injected in the putamen of the left side. It labelled the rostromedial part of the putamen and corresponding bridges of striatal tissue between the putamen and caudate nucleus (Fig. 6).

Following injection of the isotope into the most medial part of the caudate nucleus (Fig. 1) heavily labelled fibers may be successively traced through the lateral part of the caudate nucleus, the anterior limb of the internal capsule and the most medial part of the internal division of the pallidum (Figs. 1, 2). From this point the labelled striofugal fibers occupy the most medial part of the comb bundle

Fig. 1. Transverse sections through rostral part of the brain of a monkey showing site of injection of ³H-leucine in the right caudate nucleus as well as striato-pallidal and striato-nigral fibers along the dorsomedial edge of the internal division of the pallidum. ×2. C. caudate nucleus; PUT. putamen

Figs. 2 and 3. Transverse sections through the right diencephalon (2) and mes-encephalon (3) of the brain of the same monkey illustrating labelled striatonigral fibers in the medial part of the comb bundle and at the rostromedial pole of the substantia nigra, respectively. ×25, resp. ST-N striatonigral fibers; S.N. substantia nigra

Figs. 4 and 5. Transverse sections through the right substantia nigra of the same animal illustrating at low (4) and high (5) magnification labelled terminals (silver grains) in this structure. ×25 and ×400 resp. III oculomotor root fibers; S.N. substantia nigra

Fig. 6. Transverse section through right hemisphere of a monkey (macaque) brain showing site of injection of ³H-leucine at the level of the dorsomedial and rostral part of the putamen. ×4. c. caudate nucleus; put. putamen

Fig. 7. Transverse section through the rostral and central part of the external division of the right pallidum showing labelled terminals (silver grains) in this area. ×100. Dark field illumination

Fig. 8. Transverse section through the brain of the same animal illustrating labelled striatonigral fibers in the lateral part of the comb bundle. ×63. Dark-field illumination

Figs. 9 and 10. Transverse sections through the right substantia of the same animal illustrating labelled terminal endings (silver grains) in this structure. Fig. 10 corresponds to area shown in the triangle of Fig. 9. ×25 and ×63, resp. Untouched counterstained autoradiography (9) and dark-field illumination (10) s.n. substantia nigra

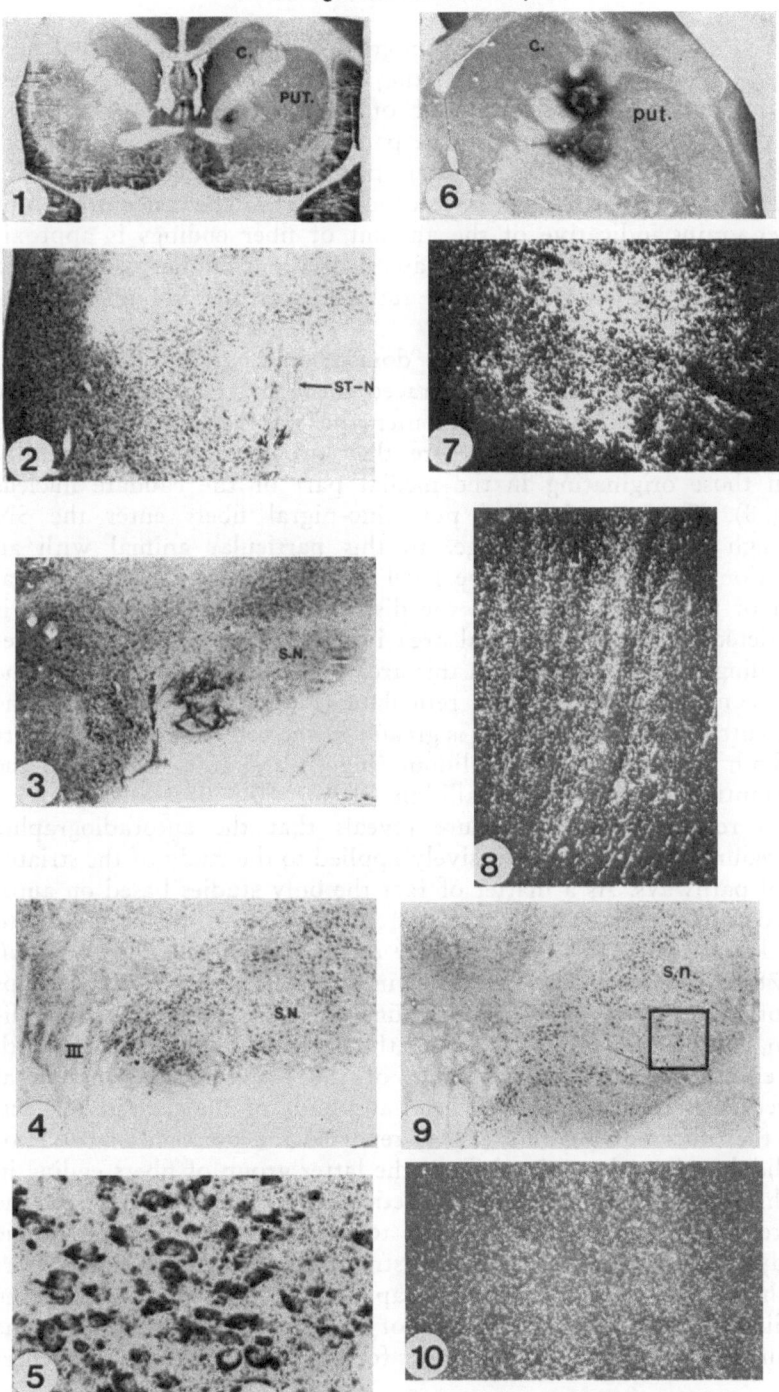

(Fig. 2) and enter the substantia nigra through its rostromedial pole (Fig. 3). Terminal labelling resulting from the injected site includes approximately the medial third of both divisions (internal and external) of the pallidum and the pars reticulata and pars compacta of the medial third of the substantia nigra (SN) (Figs. 4, 5) and in latter structure, through its rostrocaudal extent. The concentration of silver grains indicative of the amount of fiber endings is approximately equal in the medial and lateral divisions of the pallidum and in the pars compacta and pars reticulata of the SN on the corresponding side.

Following injection into the dorsomedial part of the putamen (Fig. 6) labelled fibers may be traced through both divisions of the globus pallidus. They do not enter the internal capsule but join directly the comb bundle where they are located more laterally than those originating in the medial part of the caudate nucleus (Fig. 8). Then the labelled putamino-nigral fibers enter the SN through its dorsolateral edge. In this particular animal with an injection of ³H-leucine at the level of the dorsomedial and rostral part of the putamen (Fig. 6) the distribution of the silver grains is restricted to the ventrolateral area in the rostral half of the corresponding SN (Figs. 9, 10). In this area it is evenly distributed in the pars compacta and the pars reticulata (Figs. 9, 10). Moreover the concentration of silver grains is greater in the central and rostral part of both divisions of the pallidum (Fig. 7) and it is weaker in the substantia nigra than in the pallidum (Figs. 7, 10).

A review of the literature reveals that the autoradiographic procedure has not been extensively applied to the study of the striatofugal pathways. As a matter of fact the only studies based on autoradiography and dealing with the projections of the striatum, to our knowledge, are those of *Nagy et al.* (1978) and *Tulloch et al.* (1978) in the rat and *Nauta* (1974) in the cat. The former two groups reported the presence of silver grains over the corresponding pallidum, entopenduncular nucleus and the pars reticulata and, to a much lower extent, the pars compacta of the SN following unilateral injection of ³H-leucine in the head and body of the caudate nucleus. On the other hand *Nauta* (1974) reported the presence of caudato-pallidal and caudato-nigral fibers the latter group of fibers ending in both the pars compacta and pars reticulata of the SN. Therefore the current literature does not appear to contain any autoradiographic study specically dealing with the striopallidal and strionigral fibers in the monkey. For that reason it appears appropriate to discuss the findings of this study in the light of earlier reports involving in the main silver impregnation techniques for the demonstration of degener-

ating fibers. Using such an approach *Voneida* (1960) traced degenerated axons following a lesion placed in the medial part of the
head of the caudate nucleus in the macaque. The degenerating fibers
originating from this area accumulate along the ventrolateral edge
of the internal capsule, partially end in the medial division of the
globus pallidus and proceed caudally through the basis pedunculi
before ending in the rostromedial part of the SN. According to the
author they terminate in the pars reticulata of the SN. In so far as
the course of the fibers is concerned these findings are very similar
to those obtained in this study of the squirrel and macaque brains
following injections of ^{3}H-leucine in the most medial part of the
head and body of the caudate nucleus. As a matter of fact the
documents illustrating the course of the caudato-nigral fibers as
shown with autoradiography (Figs. 1—3) could be superimposed
without any change to the corresponding microphotographs of
Voneida's paper. In this study, however, the area of the caudate
nucleus heavily labelled by ^{3}H-leucine is more extensive both dorso-
ventrally and rostrocaudally than the corresponding lesion placed
in the head of the caudate nucleus by Voneida. This most likely
explains the fact that in this material silver grains indicative of
axonal endings were concentrated in the dorsomedial area of both
divisions of the pallidum and in approximately the medial third
of the SN over the whole rostrocaudal extent of the latter structure.
Nauta (1974) also observed termination throughout the whole
rostrocaudal extent of the SN following injection of the isotope over a
large area in the central and rostral part of the caudate nucleus of
the cat. It is also interesting to note that *Cowan* and *Powell* (1966)
have reported gliosis over approximately the same areas of the
pallidum and SN following long-standing (1—4 months) lesions in
the medial part of the caudate nucleus of the macaque. On the other
hand *Szabo* (1962, 1970) also using a silver impregnation technique
has reported, in accordance with the above data, that the medial part
of the caudate nucleus projects to the medial part of both divisions
of the pallidum. However he claims that the fibers of the head of the
caudate nucleus reach the rostral SN whereas those originating in
the body of the caudate nucleus terminate in the ventrolateral area
of the SN along the basis pedunculi (*Szabo*, 1970).

  According to the same author putamino-nigral fibers which
distribute more caudally in the SN (*Szabo* 1962, 1967) would have
a tendency to terminate in the more dorsal and medial regions of the
SN (*Szabo*, 1970). These are at variance with the findings of the
present study in the monkey and those of *Nauta* (1974) in the cat
which suggest that the fibers originating in the caudate nucleus termi-

nate more medially in the SN whereas the putamino-nigral fibers terminate more laterally in this structure. There appears to exist a simple rostrocaudal and mediolateral topographical relationship between corresponding areas of the neostriatum and of the SN, as also suggested by the observation of *Cowan* and *Powell* (1966) based on the presence of gliosis in the SN following "chronic" lesions in different parts of the striatum. Our material does not permit to discuss to any great extent the dorsoventral topographical relationship between the two structures. The results of this study are also in agreement with those of *Voneida* (1960) and *Szabo* (1962, 1967, 1970) as to the effect that caudato-pallidal and putamino-pallidal fibers predominately end in the dorsomedial and the ventrolateral part of the pallidum, respectively.

Several reports based on different procedures and including reports involving autoradiography in the rat (*Nagy et al.*, 1978; *Tulloch et al.*, 1978) suggest that the strionigral fibers exclusively or predominately end in the pars reticulata of the substantia nigra. In this study, and in keeping with the findings of *Grofova* and *Rinvik* (1970) and *Nauta* (1974) in the cat, silver grains, however, were found to be equally concentrated over the neurons of the pars compacta and the pars reticulata following injection of ^{3}H-leucine either at the level of the caudate nucleus or putamen.

References

Cowan, W. M., Gottlieb, D. I., Hendrickson, A. E., Price, J. L., Woolsey, T. A.: The autoradiographic demonstration of axonal connections in the central nervous system. Brain Res. *37*, 21—51 (1972).

Cowan, W. M., Powell, T. P. S.: Strio-pallidal projection in the monkey. J. Neurol. Neurosurg. Psychiat. *29*, 426—439 (1966).

Grofova, I., Rinvik, E.: An experimental electron microscopic study on the striatonigral projection in the cat. Exp. Brain Res. *11*, 249—262 (1970).

Nagy, J. I., Carter, D. A., Fibiger, H. C.: Anterior striatal projections to the globus pallidus, entopeduncular nucleus and substantia nigra in the rat: the gaba connection. Brain Res. *158*, 15—29 (1978).

Nauta, H. J. W.: Efferent projections of the caudate nucleus, pallidal complex and subthalamic nucleus in the cat. Doctoral Dissertation, Case Western Reserve University, number 4322, p. 107 (1974).

Szabo, J.: Topical distribution of the striatal efferents in the monkey. Exp. Neurol. *5*, 21—36 (1962).

Szabo, J.: The efferent projections of the putamen in the monkey. Exp. Neurol. *19*, 463—476 (1967).

Szabo, J.: Projections from the body of the caudate nucleus in the rhesus monkey. Exp. Neurol. *27*, 1—15 (1970).

Tulloch, I. F., Arbuthnott, G. W., Wright, A. K.: Topographical organization of the striatonigral pathway revealed by anterograde and retrograde neuroanatomical tracing techniques. J. Anat. *127,* 425—441 (1978).

Voneida, T. J.: An experimental study of the course and destination of fibres, arising in the head of the caudate nucleus in the cat and monkey. J. comp. Neurol. *115,* 75—87 (1960).

Authors' address: *Louis J. Poirier,* M.D., Laboratoires de Neurobiologie, Pavillon Notre-Dame, Hôpital de l'Enfant-Jésus, 2075 de Vitré, Québec, Canada, GlJ 5B3.

Journal of Neural Transmission, Suppl. 16, 33—44 (1980)
© by Springer-Verlag 1980

Kinetics of L-DOPA Metabolism in the Caudate Nucleus of Cats with Ventrotegmental Lesions

K. G. Lloyd*, C. H. Hockmann**, Lynne Davidson, Irene J. Farley, and O. Hornykiewicz***

Clarke Institute of Psychiatry and Department of Pharmacology, University of Toronto, Toronto, Canada

Summary

Sixteen days after a unilateral lesion of the ventromedial tegmentum (VMT) of the midbrain, adult cats received an intravenous dose of L-DOPA (20 mg/kg), and the caudate nucleus from each hemisphere was removed at various time intervals thereafter. In the caudate nucleus contralateral to the VMT lesions, DA levels reached 200 % of control values within 15 min, and maintained this elevation for at least 2 hours. DA levels in the caudate nucleus ipsilateral to the VMT lesion were much lower than contralateral values; however, they were much higher than those of non-DOPA treated animals with comparable lesions. DA levels in the caudate nucleus of the lesioned hemisphere were directly related to the remaining DOPA decarboxylase activity. The striatal serotonin concentrations were unchanged after L-DOPA, but an increase in 5-hydroxyindoleacetic acid levels was observed. From these results, we conclude that, (i) in cats with nigrostriatal tract lesions after low doses of L-DOPA comparable to those given to patients with Parkinson's disease, the bulk of the newly formed DA in the caudate nucleus is contained in nigrostriatal neurons, and (ii) there exists an inverse relationship between the ability of the caudate to synthesize DA and the severity of the nigrostriatal tract lesion.

---

* Present address: Synthélabo-L.E.R.S., Department of Biology, Neuropharmacology Unit, Bagneux, France.

** Present address: School of Basic Sciences, University of Illinois, College of Medicine, Urbana, Illinois, U.S.A.

*** Present address: Institute of Biochemical Pharmacology, University of Vienna, Vienna, Austria.

Introduction

The disturbance of striatal amine metabolism found in Parkinson's disease is characterized by a severe dopamine (DA) depletion, a decrease of homovanillic acid, and a loss of DOPA decarboxylase (DOPA D) activity (*Davidson et al.*, 1971; *Hornykiewicz*, 1966, 1970; *Lloyd* and *Hornykiewicz*, 1970; *Lloyd et al.*, 1975; *Rinne et al.*, 1971, 1974). L-DOPA, the immediate precursor of DA, is the most efficacious form of treatment for Parkinson's disease, and there is good reason to believe that L-DOPA's clinical effectiveness is related to its being converted to DA in the striatum (*Calne*, 1970; *Lloyd et al.*, 1975; *Poirier et al.*, 1967).

The striatal DA deficiency of Parkinson's disease has been reproduced in different species by a number of investigators (*Goldstein et al.*, 1967; *Heller et al.*, 1969; *Hockman et al.*, 1971; *Poirier* and *Sourkes*, 1965; *Poirier et al.*, 1967; *Ungerstedt*, 1968). L-DOPA has been shown to reverse the pathophysiological concomitants of experimentally-induced Parkinsonism (*Goldstein et al.*, 1972), however, little has been done to elucidate the pharmacokinetics of L-DOPA in the animal model. In the present study, an attempt was made to assess the striatal formation of DA from L-DOPA in cats with unilateral lesions of the ventromedial tegmentum (VMT) of the midbrain inflicting damage to the nigrostriatal tract.

Methods

Forty-eight adult cats (2.3—3.5 kg of either sex) were used in this study. Anesthesia was induced with i.v. thiopental and maintained by inhalation of halothan and oxygen. Under aseptic conditions, a midline incision was made in the scalp, and a hole trephined to receive the Radionics lesioning probe. The temperature of brain tissue at the probe tip (coordinates A. 6.5; L. 2.5; D. —4), according to *Snider* and *Niemer* (1960) was slowly raised over a 100-sec period to 80 °C with a Radionics RF generator and maintained at the level for 60 sec and then allowed to return to 36 °C. The probe was then raised, Gelfoam placed over the dura, and the hole filled with a self-curing acrylic plastic. Anesthesia was discontinued while the skin was approximated and sutured. The animal received an antibiotic intramuscularly. Half of the animals were lesioned in the right hemisphere and half in the left. All animals were kept in individual cages for 16 days to permit degeneration of nigro-caudate projections (*Hockman et al.*, 1971). At this time each animal was anesthetized with sodium pentobarbital (i.p.), placed in a Kopf stereotaxic holder, and a large bilateral craniotomy was performed. The animal then received an i.v. dose of 20 mg/kg of L-DOPA. At predetermined intervals the animal received an overdose of sodium pentobarbital (i.v.). Tissue overlying the caudate nuclei was aspirated, and the caudate removed and immediately (3—4 min) frozen separately in dry ice. We found that the biochemical results did not differ between animals killed by an overdose of anesthetic prior to the removal of tissue or when tissue was removed from the anesthetized (but still living) animal. The remainder of the brain was then perfused *in situ* with a 10 %/o formalin solution. Frozen sections were stained with cresyl violet and histological examinations made of the brain stem of each animal.

The frozen striatal tissue was homogenized (5 : 1) in ice-cold isotonic dextrose. The homogenate was then divided into several aliquots. DOPA D was estimated by the formation of $^{14}CO_2$ from DL-DOPA$^{14}COOH$ as previously described (*Lloyd* and *Hornykiewicz*, 1972). The aliquot used for the determinations of L-DOPA, 3-0-methyl-DOPA, and DA was acidified with 0.4 N perchloric acid, centrifuged and applied to a Dowex column ('50WX8, 200—400 mesh) as described by *Bogdanski et al.* (1956). The effluent from the Dowex column (containing L-DOPA and 3-0-methyl-DOPA) was absorbed on alumina, and the supernatant (containing 3-0-methyl-DOPA) was applied to an amberlite column (CG-120, Type I). The 3-0-methyl-DOPA was eluted and estimated fluorimetrically as described by *Andén et al.* (1963) and *Nagatsu* and *Yamamoto* (1968). L-DOPA was then eluted from the alumina (*Nagatsu* and *Yamamoto*, 1968) and estimated fluorimetrically (*Euler* and *Floding*, 1956; *Schaepdryver*, 1958). The Dowex columns were then washed with 9.0 ml of 0.6 N HCl, and DA was eluted with 10 ml, 2.0 N HCl and estimated fluorimetrically (*Carlsson* and *Waldeck*, 1958). Recoveries for DOPA, 3-0-methyl-DOPA and DA were 63.3 ± 5.4 percent, 66.0 ± 5.3 percent and 87.8 ± 2.5 percent, respectively. The results were not corrected for recovery.

Serotonin (5-hydroxytryptamine, 5-HT) and 5-hydroxyindoleacetic acid (5-HIAA) were extracted and estimated by the adaptation of previously described procedures (*Bogdanski et al.*, 1956; *Scapagnini et al.*, 1969). Briefly, the dextrose homogenate was acidified with 0.1 N HCl, treated with zinc sulphate (16 %/o, w/v) and sodium hydroxide (5.0 N) and centrifuged ('12,000 × g × 8 min). After filtering the supernatant through glass wool, it was acidified with 2.0 N HCl and saturated with sodium chloride. The pH of the solution was adjusted to 3.5—4.0 with phosphate buffer (0.5 M, pH 7.0) containing 2 mg ascorbic acid, and the 5-HIAA extracted into chilled diethyl either. The 5-HIAA was re-extracted into phosphate buffer (0.5 M, pH 7.0), and the native fluorescence in 3.0 N HCl was measured at wavelengths of 295/543 mμ. The aqueous phase after the ether extraction was adjusted to pH 10.0 with sodium hydroxyide and stabilized by the addition of borate buffer (0.5 M, pH 10.0) and the 5-HT was extracted into 0.1 N HCl. The HCl concentration was then adjusted to 3.0 N, and the native fluorescence measured at 295/543 mμ. The recovery for 5-HT was 71.5 ± 0.8 percent and for 5-HIAA 79.9 ± 0.4 percent. The results were not corrected for recovery.

All cats were assigned to groups according to (i) the severity of the VMT lesions as determined by the DOPA D activity remaining in the caudate nucleus of the lesioned hemisphere, and (ii) an examination of stained brain stem sections. The DOPA D activity was expressed as the percentage of the mean activity in the caudate contralateral to the lesion. The remaining DOPA D activity is directly related to the severity of the destruction of the nigrostriatal DA neurons (*Hockman et al.*, 1971). The animals were divided into 3 subgroups according to the activity of DOPA D remaining in the caudate ipsilateral to the side of the VMT lesion. These 3 subgroups were: "mild" = 46—92 % DOPA D remaining; "marked" = 8.5—45 % DOPA D remaining; and "severe" = 1.5—8.4 % DOPA D remaining.

Results

Table 1 contains the results obtained from cats with unilateral VMT lesions that had not received L-DOPA. As can be seen from Table 1, there were significant differences in the levels of striatal DA between the 3 subgroups. However, the levels of striatal 5-HT did not follow the same pattern as DA, as there were no significant differences between the "severe" and "marked" groups for 5-HIAA or between "marked" and "mild" groups.

As can be seen in Table 2, 15 min after the i.v. injection of 20 mg/kg of L-DOPA, peak levels of L-DOPA were reached in the caudate nucleus of both the unlesioned and lesioned sites; these levels

Table 1. *Levels of DA, 5-HT and 5-HIAA in the caudate nucleus of non-DOPA treated cats with and without midbrain tegmental lesions of varying severity*[1]

	DA	5-HT	5-HIAA
Unlesioned[2] (100 %)	10.48 ± 0.62 (7)	0.91 ± 0.12 (8)	0.50 ± 0.08 (8)
Severe (1.5—8.4 %)	0.25 ± 0.17[3] (3)	0.18 ± 0.09[3] (3)	0.21 ± 0.09 (3)
Marked (8.5—45 %)	2.25 ± 0.87[3,4] (3)	0.40 ± 0.03[3] (3)	0.16 ± 0.06[3] (3)
Mild (46—92 %)	5.82; 4.56 (2)	0.33; 0.44 (2)	0.56; 0.15 (2)

[1] Results expressed as mean ($\mu g/g$) $\pm$ S.E.M. Number of cats in parentheses under mean. Individual values for n = 2.

[2] Degree of lesion determined by percent DOPA D activity remaining on lesioned side.

[3] $p < 0.01$ vs. unlesioned side.

[4] $p < 0.01$ vs. severely lesioned group.

Table 2. *Concentrations of L-DOPA and L-3-0-methyl-DOPA in the caudate nuclei ipsilateral and contralateral to ventrotegmental lesions in the cat*[1]

| Time after L-DOPA | Severity of lesion (DOPA D activity remaining) | | | |
	Unlesioned side (100 %)	Severe (1.5—8.4 %)	Marked (8.5—45 %)	Mild (46—92 %)
15 min	6.62 ± 1.30 (8)	—	10.51 ± 1.65 (8)	—
30 min	4.27 ± 0.36 (14)	7.10 ± 1.28[2] (3)	10.91 ± 1.40[2] (4)	5.47 ± 1.02 (7)
60 min	3.39 ± 0.45 (8)	5.64 ± 0.98 (4)	4.86 ± 1.19 (3)	1.25 (1)
120 min	1.94 ± 0.25 (4)	—	3.75; 2.98 (2)	1.59; 3.42 (2)
240 min	0.84 ± 0.34 (8)	0.66 ± 0.66 (3)	0.70 ± 0.70 (3)	0.82 (1)

[1] All values expressed as mean (μg/g) ± S.E.M. Number of animals in parentheses.

[2] $p < 0.02$ vs. unlesioned side.

declined with an apparent half-life of about 60 min, indicating that VMT lesions did not alter the half-life of L-DOPA in the caudate.

However, despite the unchanged half-life of L-DOPA in the caudate ipsilateral to the VMT lesion, L-DOPA concentrations at 30 min post injection were significantly higher ($p < 0.02$) than the contralateral caudate (Table 2).

In contrast to L-DOPA, 3-0-methyl-DOPA levels were not detectable (*i.e.* < 0.40 μg/g) in the caudate until at least 120 min after administration of L-DOPA and then were consistently demonstrable only in the caudate contralateral to the lesion (0.92 ± 0.54 μg/g, n = 4 at 120 min; 1.39 ± 0.53 μg/g, n = 8 at 240 min).

As shown in Table 3, DA levels in the control caudate (*i.e.* contralateral to VMT lesions) were greatly increased after L-DOPA injections. This increase was maximal at 15 min and was maintained at that level until at least 120 min after the injection of the drug. A decline in DA levels was observed at 240 min. Compared with endogenous DA levels the peak DA levels reached 230 % after i.v. L-DOPA, 20 mg/kg.

In the caudate ipsilateral to the VMT lesion the DA levels after L-DOPA were inversely proportional to the severity of the lesion. This is evident from Table 3, which shows that the levels of DA at 30,

Table 3. *Concentration of DA in the caudate nucleus, ipsilateral and contralateral to ventrotegmental lesions in the cat*[1]

Severity of lesion (in parentheses: % of DOPA D)	Time after L-DOPA (min)				
	15	30	60	120	240
Unlesioned hemisphere (100 %)	21.80 ± 2.64 (8)	20.16 ± 2.19 (14)	17.68 ± 2.05 (8)	24.36 ± 3.42 (4)	14.69 ± 1.17 (8)
Severe (1.5—8.4 %)	—	1.37; <0.01 (2)	1.59^2 ± 0.91 (4)	—	2.11^2 ± 0.87 (3)
Marked (8.5—45 %)	5.06^2 ± 0.67 (8)	4.47^2 ± 2.34 (4)	$8.13^{2, 3}$ ± 0.70 (4)	4.66; 5.29 (2)	6.75^2 ± 2.29 (3)
Mild (46—92 %)	7.59 (1)	15.52 ± 3.48 (7)	17.04 (1)	21.94; 16.49 (2)	8.10 (1)

[1] Results expressed as mean (μg/g) ± S.E.M. Number of animals in parentheses.
[2] $p < 0.01$ vs. unlesioned hemisphere.
[3] $p < 0.01$ vs. severely lesioned groups.

60 and 120 min after L-DOPA were directly related to the absolute DOPA D levels in the caudate. In the animals with "severe" VMT lesions DA formation in the ipsilateral caudate after L-DOPA administration was demonstrable only in 5 of the 9 animals examined. At all time intervals the DA levels in these animals were much lower than for any other group.

In each of the three lesioned groups, the 5-HT levels in the caudate ipsilateral to the VMT lesion were significantly lower, but did not parallel the decrease in DOPA D activity. L-DOPA injections did not have any apparent effect on the 5-HT concentrations in the caudate of either the non-lesioned or the lesioned hemisphere (Table 4).

In contrast to 5-HT, the 5-HIAA levels were increased in the control caudates of L-DOPA treated animals when compared with non-DOPA treated cats (Table 4). This increase in 5-HIAA was statistically significant ($p < 0.05$ or less) for all time intervals after L-DOPA. In the caudate of the hemisphere ipsilateral to the VMT lesion of the "severely" and "markedly" lesioned groups, the absolute levels of 5-HIAA in response to L-DOPA (as compared to non-L-DOPA treated animals with lesions of equal severity) was greater.

However, due to the wide range of single values in the lesioned animals these 5-HIAA increases were statistically significant for only a few selected time intervals (see Table 4).

Table 4. *Concentrations of 5-HT and 5-HIAA in the caudate nuclei ipsilateral and contralateral to ventrotegmental lesions in the cat*[1]

Time after L-DOPA (min)	Unlesioned hemisphere		Severe (1.4—8.4 %)		Marked (8.5—45 %)		Mild (46—92 %)	
	5-HT	5-HIAA	5-HT	5-HIAA	5-HT	5-HIAA	5-HT	5-HIAA
0	0.91 ±0.12 (8)	0.50 ±0.08 (8)	0.18[3] ±0.09 (3)	0.21 ±0.03 (3)	0.40[3] ±0.03 (3)	0.16[3] ±0.06 (3)	0.33; 0.44 (2)	0.56; 0.15 (2)
15	0.93 ±0.06 (8)	0.67 ±0.05 (8)	—	—	0.54 ±0.10 (8)	0.31[5] ±0.04 (8)	—	—
30	0.84 ±0.06 (14)	0.79[2] ±0.08 (14)	0.25[5] ±0.03 (3)	1.36 ±0.96 (3)	0.33[4] ±0.06 (4)	0.39[4] ±0.09 (4)	0.43[5] ±0.07 (7)	0.84 ±0.17 (7)
60	0.94 ±0.08 (8)	0.95[3] ±0.08 (8)	0.28[5] ±0.11 (4)	0.39[5] ±0.04 (4)	0.31[5] ±0.07 (3)	0.96 ±0.36 (3)	0.82 (1)	1.51 (1)
120	0.67 ±0.07 (5)	0.83[2] ±0.10 (4)	—	—	0.09; 0.18 (2)	0.15; 0.33 (2)	0.31; 1.14 (2)	1.59; 3.42 (2)
240	0.85 ±0.07 (8)	1.14[3] ±0.07 (8)	0.21[5] ±0.02 (3)	0.50[5] ±0.08 (2)	0.39; 0.59 (2)	0.92; 0.96 (2)	0.82 (1)	2.10 (1)

[1] Values expressed as mean (μg/g) ± S.E.M. Number of animals in parentheses.
[2] $p < 0.05$ vs. 0 time (Table 1).
[3] $p < 0.01$ vs. 0 time.
[4] $p < 0.05$ vs. unlesioned hemisphere.
[5] $p < 0.01$ vs. unlesioned hemisphere.

Discussion

The most significant result of our study is the demonstration that in the caudate ipsilateral to a VMT lesion the peak concentrations of DA attained, after i.v. administration of 20 mg/kg, were directly related to the severity of the VMT lesion. Thus, in "severely" lesioned animals, the peak DA level attained after L-DOPA was only 10 % of the control value, and probably did not occur until 2—4 hours after the drug; in animals with "marked" lesions, the maximum DA levels were reached 60 min after L-DOPA, being at that time about 40 % of the control value; and in the "mildly" lesioned animals, the caudate DA changes after L-DOPA approximated the changes seen in the control caudates.

The increase in DA levels in the caudate of the control side after i.v. L-DOPA was quantitatively similar to that reported for the cat by *Dagirmajian et al.* (1963) and *Poirier et al.* (1967). In the present experiments, the increase was maximal within 15 min and remained at that level for at least 2 hours; 4 hours after the injection the levels were still increased by about 50 %.

The lesion-dependent decrease in DA synthesis from exogenous L-DOPA as observed in the present study is in marked contrast to a study using rats with 6-OHDA which showed no difference from controls in DA formation after the administration of L-DOPA (*Lytle et al.*, 1972). In the latter study, the 6-OHDA lesion of the nigrostriatal DA path (60—65 % reduction) was likely too mild, and is comparable to our results in animals with "mild lesions". This suggestion as well as the very high dose of L-DOPA (200 mg/kg) used by the investigators (*Lytle et al.*, 1972) most probably accounts for the formation of large amounts of DA, similar in magnitude to that of control animals. In this context, it is interesting to note that, in the present experiments (Table 3) cats with "mild" lesions formed 8 to 10 times more DA than did animals with severe lesions and 30 to 120 min after L-DOPA these levels could not be distinguished from those in the contralateral (*i.e.* unlesioned hemisphere) caudate.

Also, in some species (*e.g.* the rat) a blood-brain barrier exists for L-DOPA at least partly in the form of a capillary decarboxylase (*Bertler et al.*, 1966; *Constantinidis et al.*, 1967; *De La Torre*, 1972; *Owman* and *Rosengren*, 1967). This could contribute to the considerable formation of DA from L-DOPA (*Lytle et al.*, 1972) after 6-OHDA treatment in the rat (which would leave the capillary decarboxylase intact). However, such a barrier for L-DOPA apparently is not a critical factor in the cat as indicated by the previous studies (*Langelier et al.*, 1972; *Dowson*, 1973) and by the present findings that severe VMT lesions can almost completely eliminate DOPA decarboxylase activity in the cat caudate nucleus.

Our results from the "severely" lesioned animals are in general agreement with those of *Poirier et al.* (1967) who showed that in cats DA formation after L-DOPA administration was greatly decreased in the striatum ipsilateral to extensive brain stem lesions. The present elucidation of an inverse relationship between the degree of damage to the nigrostriatal tract and striatal DA formation after injected

L-DOPA demonstrates that this DA synthesis takes place within cells that normally synthesize and store DA. Additionally, in doses of 20 mg/kg (present study) to 70 mg/kg (*Poirier et al.*, 1967) the fate of the injected L-DOPA (at least in the striatum) is similar to that of the endogenous DA precursor. In our earlier experiments, we showed that DOPA D activity in the caudate of the lesioned hemisphere bears a direct relationship to the severity of the lesion (*Hockman et al.*, 1971). In the present experiments, DOPA D activity also proved to be a valid index of the severity of nigrostriatal tract damage, as judged by the ability of the caudate to form DA from endogenous L-DOPA.

The half-life of L-DOPA (60 min) in the caudate of our cats was similar to that in the rat (*Bartholini* and *Pletscher*, 1968) and was unaffected by VMT lesion. The low concentrations of 3-0-methyl-DOPA that appeared after the administration of L-DOPA precluded the determination of its half-life.

The decrease in 5-HT following VMT lesions was probably caused by an interruption of the more medially located 5-HT fibers (*Hockman et al.*, 1971; *Poirier et al.*, 1967). The observation that L-DOPA administration did not alter striatal 5-HT levels is not in agreement with earlier reports in non-lesioned animals (*Bartholini et al.*, 1968; *Everett* and *Borcherding*, 1970; *Karobath et al.*, 1971). However, in our study, a distinctly lower dose of L-DOPA was utilized. Despite the absence of an effect of L-DOPA on brain 5-HT, the 5-HIAA levels were markedly elevated. This increase occurred in the caudates of both hemispheres suggesting that a dose of L-DOPA even as low as 20 mg/kg interferes with the steady state of the striatal 5-HT system.

A comparison between the neurochemistry of the present animal model, and that of patients dying with Parkinson's disease (average caudate DOPA D activity 15 % of control) (*Lloyd et al.*, 1975); 5-HT decrease by 40 % or less (*Bernheimer et al.*, 1961) places the Parkinsonian patients in the lower range of the experimental group with "marked" lesions. The disproportionately lower striatal DA levels in Parkinson's disease are likely due to a compensatory over-activity of the remaining DA neurons in response to this chronic condition (*Hornykiewicz*, 1966; *Lloyd et al.*, 1975); this is in contrast to the comparatively acute state present in the lesioned animals. Accordingly, (i) the decrease in DA in the caudate of non-DOPA treated Parkinsonism (*Lloyd et al.*, 1975) is very similar to that presently observed for the ipsilateral caudate in non-DOPA treated marked-severe lesioned cats; (ii) a number of Parkinsonian patients treated chronically with doses of L-DOPA (1 g single oral dose) comparable to the 20 mg/kg (i.v.) dose of our cats, had DA levels in the striatum approaching the control range (*Lloyd et al.*, 1975); this is similar to the behaviour of our cats with "marked" lesions. In addition, as in our cats, in Parkinsonian patients L-DOPA does not influence the somewhat subnormal (*Bernheimer et al.*, 1961; *Rinne and Sonninen*, 1972) 5-HT levels in the brain; however, there is a distinct elevation of brain 5-HIAA (*Rinne* and *Sonninen*, 1972). In contrast to our cats, Parkinsonian patients exhibit high striatal concentrations of 3-0-methyl-DOPA within 2.5 hours after ingestion (*Lloyd et al.*, 1975). However, this difference could be due to the formation of a 3-0-methyl-DOPA pool in patients during long-term L-DOPA therapy (*Kuruma et al.*, 1970).

In conclusion, it seems justified to say that, in many major aspects, the experimental model of cats with VMT lesions represents an accurate reflection of the neurochemistry of the Parkinsonian condition.

Acknowledgement

This study was generously supported by a research grant from the Playfair Fund of the University of Toronto and by the Clarke Institute of Psychiatry and by Eaton Laboratories, Norwich, New York, U.S.A.

References

Andén, N.-E., Roos, B.-E., Werdinius, B.: On the occurrence of homovanillic acid in brain and cerebrospinal fluid and its determination by a fluorimetric method. Life Sciences 2, 448—458 (1968).

Bartholini, G., Pletscher, A.: Cerebral accumulation and metabolism of ^{14}C-L-DOPA after selective inhibition of peripheral decarboxylase. J. Pharmacol. Exp. Ther. *161*, 14—20 (1968).

Bartholini, G., Da Prada, M., Pletscher, A.: Decrease of cerebral 5-hydroxytryptamine by 3, 4-dihydroxyphenylalanine after inhibition of extracerebral decarboxylase. J. Pharm. Pharmac. 20, 219—229 (1968).

Bernheimer, H., Birkmayer, W., Hornykiewicz, O.: Verteilung des 5-Hydroxy-tryptamin (Serotonin) im Gehirn des Menschen und sein Verhalten bei Patienten mit Parkinson-Syndrom. Klin. Wsch. *39*, 1056—1059 (1961).

Bertler, A., Falck, B., Owman, Ch., Rosengren, E.: The localization of monoaminergic blood-brain mechanisms. Pharmacol. Revs. *18*, 369—385 (1966).

Bogdanski, D. F., Pletscher, A., Brodie, A., Brodie, B. B., Udenfriend, S.: Identification and assay of serotonin in brain. J. Pharmacol. Exp. Ther. *117*, 82—88 (1956).

Calne, D. B.: Parkinsonism. London: Arnold. 1970.

Carlsson, A., Waldeck, B.: A fluorimetric method for the determination of dopamine (3-hydroxytyramine). Acta Physiol. Scand. *44*, 293—298 (1958).

Constantinidis, J., De La Torre, J. C., Tissot, R., Geissbühler, F.: La barrière capillaire pour la L-DOPA dans le cerveau et les differents organes. Psychopharmacologia *15*, 75—87 (1969).

Dagirmanjian, R., Laverty, R., Mantegazzini, P., Sharman, D. F., Vogt, M.: Chemical and physiological changes produced by arterial infusion of dihydroxyphenylalanine into one cerebral hemisphere of the cat. J. Neurochem. *10*, 117—182 (1963).

Davidson, L., Lloyd, K. G., Dankova, J., Hornykiewicz, O.: L-DOPA treatment in Parkinson's disease: effect on dopamine and related substances in discrete brain regions. Experientia *27*, 1048—1049 (1971).

De La Torre, J. C.: The blood-brain barrier for L-DOPA in the hypothalamus. J. Neurol. Sci. *12*, 77—93 (1971).

Dowson, J. H.: Animal models for an enzymic blood-brain barrier mechanism for therapeutically administered L-DOPA. Life Sciences *13*, 23—29 (1973).

Euler, U. S. Von, Floding, I.: Diagnosis of pheochromocytoma by fluorimetric estimation of adrenaline and noradrenaline in urine. Scand. J. Clin. Lab. Invest. *8*, 288—295 (1956).

Everett, G. M., Borcherding, J. W.: L-DOPA: Effect on concentrations of 5-hydroxytryptamine in brains of mice. Science *168*, 849—850 (1970).

Goldstein, M., Anagnoste, B., Owen, W. S., Battista, A. F.: The effects of ventromedial tegmental lesions on the disposition of dopamine in the caudate nucleus of the monkey. Brain Research *4*, 298—300 (1967).

Goldstein, M., Anagnoste, B., Battista, A. F., Nakatani, S., Ogawa, M.: Biochemical aspects of experimentally induced parkinsonism. Neurotransmitters Res. Publ., A.R.N.M.D. *50*, 434—437 (1972).

Heller, A., Bhatnagar, R. K., Moore, R. Y.: Selective neuronal control of telencephalic monoamines and enzymes involved in their biosynthesis. In: Progress in Neurogenetics (*Barbeau, A., Brunette, J. R.,* eds.), pp. 283—288. Amsterdam: Excerpta Medica. 1969.

Hockman, C. H., Lloyd, K. G., Farley, I. G., Hornykiewicz, O.: Experimental midbrain lesions: neurochemical comparison between the animal model and Parkinson's disease. Brain Research *35*, 613—618 (1971).

Hornykiewicz, O.: Dopamine (3-hydroxytyramine) and brain function. Pharmacol. Rev. *18*, 925—962 (1966).

Hornykiewicz, O.: Physiological, biochemical and pathological background of levodopa and possibilities for the future. Neurology *20*, 1—5 (1970).

Karobath, M., Diaz, J. L., Huttunen, M. O.: The effect of L-DOPA on the concentrations of tryptophan, tyrosine and serotonin in rat brain. Europ. J. Pharmacol. *14*, 393—396 (1971).

Kuruma, I., Bartholini, G., Pletscher, A.: L-DOPA induced accumulation of 3-0-methyl-DOPA in brain and heart. Europ. J. Pharmacol. *10*, 189—192 (1970).

Langelier, P., Parent, A., Poirier, L. J.: Decarboxylase activity of the brain capillary walls and parenchyma in the rat, cat and monkey. Brain Research *45*, 622—629 (1972).

Lloyd, K. G., Hornykiewicz, O.: Parkinson's disease: Activity of L-DOPA decarboxylase in discrete brain regions. Science 170, 1212—1213 (1970).

Lloyd, K. G., Hornykiewicz, O.: Occurrence and distribution of aromatic L-amino acid (L-DOPA) decarboxylase in the human brain. J. Neurochem. 19, 1549—1559 (1972).

Lloyd, K. G., Davidson, L., Hornykiewicz, O.: The neurochemistry of Parkinson's disease: effect of L-DOPA therapy. J. Pharmacol. Exp. Ther. 195, 453—464 (1975).

Lytle, L. D., Hurko, D., Romero, J. A., Cottman, K., Leehey, D., Wurtman, R. J.: The effects of 6-hydroxydopamine pretreatment on the accumulation of DOPA and dopamine in brain and peripheral organs following L-DOPA administration. J. Neural Transm. 33, 63—71 (1972).

Owman, Ch., Rosengren, E.: Dopamine formation in brain capillaries and enzymic blood-brain barrier mechanism. J. Neurochem. 14, 547—550 (1967).

Nagatsu, T., Yamamoto, T.: Fluorescence assay of tyrosine hydroxylase activity in tissue homogenate. Experientia 24, 1183—1184 (1968).

Poirier, L. J., Sourkes, T. L.: Influence of the substantia nigra on the catecholamine content of the striatum. Brain 88, 181—192 (1965).

Poirier, L. J., Singh, P., Sourkes, T. L., Boucher, R.: Effect of amines precursors on the concentration of striatal dopamine and serotonin in cats with and without unilateral brainstem. Brain Research 6, 954—966 (1967).

Rinne, U. K., Sonninen, V.: Brain catecholamines and their metabolites in parkinsonian patients. Arch. Neurol. 28, 107—110 (1972).

Rinne, U. K., Sonninen, V., Hyyppa, M.: Effect of L-DOPA on brain monoamines and their metabolites in Parkinson's disease. Life Sciences I, 10, 549—557 (1971).

Rinne, U. K., Sonninen, V., Rickkinen, P., Laaksonen, H.: Dopaminergic nervous transmission in Parkinson's disease. Med. Biol. 52, 208—217 (1974).

Scapagnini, U., Vandenbroeck, R., Schaepdryver, A. D. de: Simultaneous estimation of 5-hydroxytryptamine and 5-hydroxy-indole-3-acetic acid in rat brain. Biochem. Pharmacol. 18, 938—940 (1969).

Schaepdryver, A. D. de: Differential fluorimetric estimation of adrenaline and noradrenaline in urine. Arch. Int. Pharmacodyn. 115, 233—245 (1958).

Snider, R. S., Niemer, W. T.: A stereotaxic atlas of the cat brain. Chicago: Univ. of Chicago Press. 1960.

Ungerstedt, U.: 6-Hydroxydopamine induced degeneration of central monoamine neurons. Europ. J. Pharmacol. 5, 107—110 (1968).

Authors' address: Dr. K. G. Lloyd, Chief, Department of Neuropharmacology, L.E.R.S., 31, Avenue P. V. Couturier, F-92220 Bagneux, France.

Journal of Neural Transmission, Suppl. 16, 45—51 (1980)
© by Springer-Verlag 1980

Spiroperidol Binding in the Human Caudate Nucleus

M. H. Winkler, S. Berl, W. O. Whetsell, jr., and M. D. Yahr

The Clinical Center for Parkinson Research, Department of Neurology, The Mount Sinai School of Medicine, City University of New York, New York, N.Y., U.S.A.

With 2 Figures

Summary

The displacement of spiroperidol binding by the optical isomers of butaclamol in synaptosomal preparations of the caudate nucleus obtained from parkinsonians and non-parkinsonians at post mortem were investigated. A group of spiroperidol binding sites found in the non-parkinsonians was less strongly expressed or absent in analogous tissue of the parkinsonian. The significance of these findings in relation to Parkinson's disease and its treatment are discussed.

It is now well established that a deficiency of dopamine (DA) in the human striatum correlates with the major clinical manifestations of parkinsonism—namely, motor dysfunction. However, the fundamental mechanism by which DA mediates motor processes and the neural circuits impaired by its loss, are far from clear. In part, this reflects our lack of precise information concerning the intrinsic structure of the striatum particularly the nature of its synaptic transactions. A number of correlative studies are now on-going in our laboratories relative to the morphologic, physiologic and biochemical characteristics of the human striatum. We wish herein to report one aspect of this study.

It now seems probable that the binding of a particular neurotransmitter in the CNS seldom, if ever, involves only first order binding to one homogeneous set of sites. In a recently completed study of GABA binding to a synaptic membrane suspension prepared from rat brain our data indicated that either a very complex binding by a single set of sites occurs or that binding by several independent sets of GABA receptor sites or both, are operative [1]. It has been possible to differentiate between complex binding by a single set of sites as opposed to several sets of sites by chemically inactivating one homogeneous set. On the basis of detailed binding curves Creese, et al. [2] postulated at least two sets of binding sites for dopamine were evident in crude rat brain homogenates. Similar conclusions have been reached as a result of the discovery of adenylate cyclase activating and adenylate cyclase independent dopamine receptors [3] and on the basis of differential drug effects [4, 5]. Data published by Hartley and Seeman [6] are consistent with the existence of 2 sets of sites in bovine caudate. The fact that a single molecular species, spiroperidol, may bind primarily to dopaminergic sites in the striatum [7] and serotonergic sites in the frontal cortex [8] suggests that existence of flexibility and/or multi-specificity in individual receptor sites themselves.

A racemic mixture of the butaclamols is a potent competitive inhibitor of spiroperidol binding; the (+)isomer has been found to be a thousand times more active than its enantiomers in the striatum and several hundred times more active in the frontal cortex [9]. Most of the studies of butaclamol displacement of spiroperidol have related to the highest affinity binding sites: a set or a group of sets which appears to saturate below 2 nM free spiroperidol [9]. On the basis of the rapidly accumulating evidence for multiple sets of sites and since the stimulated release of neurotransmitter into the synaptic cleft may result in the post-synaptic membrane being exposed to high concentrations of transmitter [10, 11] we undertook a search for, and the study of, lower affinity sets of sites. We herein report on the displacement of spiroperidol binding by the optical isomers of butaclamol from synaptic membrane preparations (SMP) of the caudate nucleus obtained from human post mortem patients with parkinsonism and normal controls. Displacement was affected subsequent to the equilibration of the membranes with 2 to 16 nM spiroperidol.

Methods

Briefly, tissues for the studies were obtained from the caudates of parkinsonian and non-parkinsonian post-mortem brains. Those with Parkinson's disease had been under the care of one of us (MDY) had been treated with levodopa and carbidopa until intercurrent disease prevented its administration. No patient had received these agents within 5 days of their demise. The brains were removed within 6 hours of death and maintained at $-80\,°C$ until required. The same region of caudate nucleus was dissected from each brain at $-12\,°C$ in a cryostat. Synaptic membranes were prepared by slight modification of procedures previously described [12]. Each caudate specimen was homogenized in pH 7.4 sucrose-tris-EDTA buffer (10 ml/gm wet weight). After low speed centrifugation the pellet was discarded and supernatant again centrifuged at $12,500 \times g$ for 8 min. The resulting pellet was resuspended in 10 ml of a 3 % Ficoll-buffer solution. This suspension was carefully layered over 20 ml of a 6 % Ficoll-buffer solution and centrifuged at $10,800 \times g$ for 30 min. Both layers were separated from the mitochondrial pellet, combined with a superficial wash and the resulting suspension diluted 4-fold with distilled water. After standing for 20 min at room temperature it was centrifuged at $12,500 \times g$ and the pellet resuspended in distilled water. Samples were taken for protein determinations and the suspension then divided into aliquots and frozen at $-20\,°C$. When required, the appropriate number of aliquots were thawed, repelleted and resuspended in buffer "A" (15 mM tris, 5 mM EDTA, 1.1 mM ascorbate, pH 7.4). The binding of spiroperidol was determined by initial equilibrations in 16×125 Nalgene tubes of six portions (0.2 mg protein each) of the synaptic membrane preparation with each ^{3}H-spiroperidol concentration. Equilibration tubes contained 1.8 ml of buffer A, 0.1 ml of the desired quantity of ^{3}H-spiroperidol and 0.1 ml of the SMP suspension. Equilibrations were continued for 20 minutes at room temperature with gentle agitation. After this period of 20 μl portions of 2.5 μM (+)butaclamol were added to three of each set of six tubes and the same amount of (—)butaclamol added to the remaining three tubes. Equilibrations were continued for another 20 minutes after which time the tubes were centrifuged at $49,000 \times g$ and 4 $°C$ for 1 hour. The pellets were superficially washed twice with cold distilled water and transferred to 10 ml of a liquid scintillation fluid (Scintiverse, Fisher Scientific, New York). Radioactivity was determined in a Packard Tri-Carb liquid scintillation counter.

Results

Data obtained in a representative experiment utilizing membranes prepared from a non-parkinsonian caudate is presented in Fig. 1. Curves 1 and 2 describe, respectively, the retention of radioactivity after the addition of (+)- or (—)butaclamol. The most significant feature of this set of curves is that they cross and as a result the difference curve, curve 3, changes sign. This observation is most easily reconciled with the assumption that two or more sets of spiroperidol binding sites are being expressed by the homogenate and that at least one set of sites binds (—)butaclamol more avidly than it binds its enantiomer.

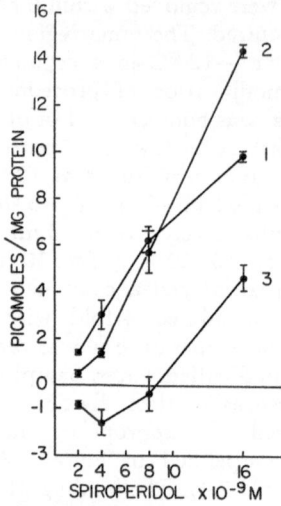

Fig. 1. Residual retentions of ^{3}H-spiroperidol by synaptic membrane pellets formed from a non-parkinsonian caudate after displacement with 25 nM (+) (curve I) or (—) (curve 2) butaclamol. Curve three is the difference between curves 1 and 2. The vertical lines of curves 1 and 2 give the range of triplicate determinations. The vertical lines superimposed on curve 3 represent standard deviations. Displacements are plotted as a function of the free ^{3}H-spiroperidol concentrations at equilibrium

Discussion

These results supplement previous findings in that: (1) we are herein reporting observations made with an SMP which has been equilibrated with concentrations of spiroperidol far in excess of those reported in the previous investigations cited, and (2) we are investigating displacement rather than inhibition. In general, displacement and inhibition will not be identical if equilibration is slow or if a conformational change accompanied binding. Work, in progress, in our laboratory indicates that the result of binding studies on bovine caudate SMP's are not independent of the time at which an excess of unlabelled spiroperidol is added when an excess of cold spiroperidol is used to define non-specific binding.

The fact that studies in other laboratories have indicated saturation of the very high affinity sites which they have investigated at lower free spiroperidol concentration together with the results reported above signified that we are dealing with a different group of sites. These sites are of lower affinity and apparently capable of binding several hundred times as much ligand. The previously cited study *Hartley* and *Seeman* [6] is consistent with the existence of two sets of spiroperidol binding sites in bovine caudate SMP. One set, expressed primarily after equilibration with higher (nanomolar) concentrations of spiroperidol, has a greater capacity than the higher affinity set.

A parallel study repeated with an homogenate prepared from a parkinsonian caudate does not yield a difference curve which is negative or zero over any portion of the concentration range herein reported. This difference between parkinsonian and non-parkinsonian brains from patients of approximately the same age has been confirmed on caudate homogenates from 6 parkinsonians, Fig. 2 a and from 3 non-parkinsonians, Fig. 2 b (two ALS, and one caudate from a

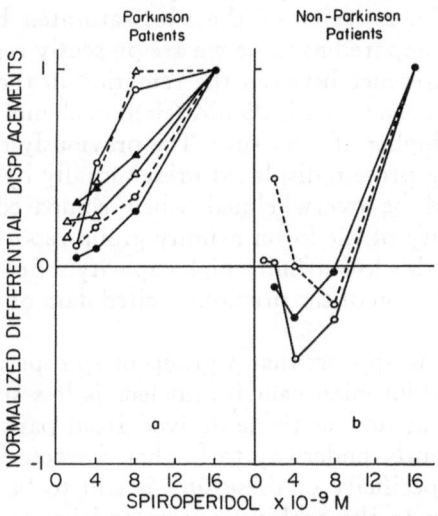

Fig. 2. Summary of the differences in displacements by (+)butaclamol minus the displacements by (—)butaclamol as a function of free ^{3}H-spiroperidol concentrations at equilibrium. The data is plotted as a fraction of the differential displacements from membrane pellets which had been previously equilibrated with 16 nM spiroperidol, *a* parkinsonian, *b* non-parkinsonian tissue

patient with no known neurological disease). Additionally, sufficient caudate was available from a Huntington's brain and from another non-parkinsonian brain to do determinations in triplicate, at 8 nM spiroperidol. It was found again for preparations made from non-parkinsonian derived tissue that (—)butaclamol displaces a portion of the spiroperidol bound at 8 nM more efficiently than does its enantiomer. Thus, in every instance the non-parkinsonian tissue yielded a preparation for which (—)butaclamol was equal to, or a more efficient displacer of some concentration of ^{3}H-spiroperidol than was (+)butaclamol. This was never true for the six parkinsonian tissues studied. *Hoss et al.* [13] had reported that both enantiomers of butaclamol were of equal potency in displacing apomorphine from rat brain membranes, but we are not aware of any previous reports of the (—)isomer being the more potent of the two.

The relevance of this low affinity high capacity group of binding sites may warrant more attention than is generally accorded them. It has been estimated that after transmitter release into a synaptic cleft the concentration of transmitter (to which post-synaptic membranes are exposed) may be high [10, 11] and therefore the behavior of membranes in the presence of high concentrations of specifically, bound ligands may more adequately represent an *in vivo* situation.

Because of the capacity of the sites saturated below 2 nM free spiroperidol as compared to those we are presently reporting, negative value for the difference between the retention in the presence of the enantiomer may occur even if 25 nM (+)butaclamol totally displaces the ligand from higher affinity sites. The previously reported capacity of 250 fmoles/mg protein displaced preferentially by the (+)enantiomer [14] would be overwhelmed when compared to the several picomolar capacity of the lower affinity group reported in this paper. The existence of this low affinity high capacity set can also be derived from an extrapolation of the previously cited data of *Hartley* and *Seeman* [6].

In summary, it appears that a group of spiroperidol binding sites found in nonparkinsonian caudate nucleus is less strongly expressed or absent in the analogous tissue derived from parkinsonian sources. Studies are currently underway to further characterize these sites. At this point, the specificity of these sites is still to be determined as is their relationship to the parkinson state and its treatment. Conceivably, their loss may play a role in the etiology of parkinsonism.

Acknowledgements

The authors wish to express their gratitude to Ms. Ellen Manos and Ms. Ellen Braunstein for their invaluable assistance.

This work was support in party by the Clinical Center for Research in Parkinson's and Allied Diseases, NIH Grant NS-11631-06.

References

[1] *Winkler, M. H., Nicklas, W. J., Berl, S.:* J. Neurochem. *32*, 79—84 (1979).

[2] Creese, I., Burt, D. R. S., Snyder, S. H.: Life Sci. 17, 993—1002 (1975).

[3] Schwarcz, R., Kjell, F., Agnati, L. F., Gustafson, J.: Life Sci. 23, 465—470 (1978).

[4] Titeler, M., Weinreich, P., Sinclair, D., Seeman, P.: Proc. Nat. Acad. Sci. 75, 1153—1156 (1978).

[5] Beld, A. J., Kiujer, B., Rodriguez de Miranda, J. F., Wonterese, A. C.: Life Sci. 28, 489 (1978).

[6] Hartley, E. J., Seeman, P.: Life Sci. 23, 513—518 (1978).

[7] Leysen, J. E., Gommeren, W., Laduron, P. M.: Biochem. Pharmac. 27, 307—316 (1978).

[8] Leysen, J. E., Neimegeers, C. J. E., Tollenacre, J. P., Laduron, P. M.: Nature 272, 168—171 (1978).

[9] Leysen, J. E., Gommeren, W.: Life Sci. 23, 447—452 (1978).

[10] Jonsson, G., Sachs, C.: European J. Pharmac. 16, 55 (1971).

[11] Symes, A. L., Lal, S., Sourkes, T. L.: J. Pharm. Pharmacol. 29, 44—45 (1977).

[12] Puszkin, S., Nicklas, W. J., Berl, S.: J. Neurochem. 19, 1319—1333 (1972).

[13] Hoss, W., Reese, J. H., Smiley, C.: J. Neurosci. Res. 3, 257—266 (1977).

[14] Reisine, T. D., Fields, J. Z., Bird, E. D., Spokes, E., Yomomura, H. I.: Comm. Psychopharm. 2, 75—84 (1978).

Authors' address: Dr. M. D. Yahr, Professor and Chairman, Department of Neurology, The Mount Sinai School of Medicine, 100th Street at Fifth Avenue, New York, NY 10029, U.S.A.

Journal of Neural Transmission, Suppl. 16, 53—67 (1980)
© by Springer-Verlag 1980

Quantitative Dissection of Human Brain Areas: Relevance to Transmitter Analyses

St. Wuketich, P. Riederer, K. Jellinger, and L. Ambrozi

Department of Pathology, Lainz-Hospital, Wien, Ludwig Boltzmann-Institute of
Clinical Neurobiology, Lainz-Hospital, Wien, Austria

Summary

Comparison of the fresh weights of whole brains and of five quantitatively dissected subcortical nuclei (caudate n., putamen, globus pallidus,
amygdala, n. ruber) were performed between 11 cases of Parkinson's disease
(76.5 ± 1.85 years), 4 cases of Huntington's chorea (63.2 ± 1.9 years) and
17 age-matched controls without neurological disorders (71.53 ± 0.26 years).
The fresh weights of these brain loci and the concentrations of dopamine
(DA), norepinephrine (NE) and serotonin (5-HT) in controls and parkinsonian brains were compared. The average weight of parkinsonian brain
was 1136.2 ± 100.1 g and was 1181.6 ± 154.8 g for controls, with no
difference in the weights of the lenticular nuclei between these two groups,
while in Huntington's chorea there was significant reduction of the whole
brain weight (84.3 % of controls) and of the caudate n. and putamen (47.4
and 43.3 %). The gl. pallidus was less severely reduced in Huntington's
chorea (73.2 %), while the weights of the amygdala and n. ruber were
similar for the three groups. Comparison of the absolute and relative concentrations of monoamines in the 5 dissected nuclei was performed.
Parkinsonian brains showed a severe reduction of DA in the caudate n.,
putamen and gl. pallidus (5 %, 10 % and 12 % of controls), and n. ruber
(11 % of controls) of NE in n. ruber (33 %), caudate n. and putamen (45 %
and 55 %) and of 5-HT in gl. pallidus and amygdala (30 %), caudate n.
(44 %) and putamen (57 % of controls), and n. ruber (64 % of controls).
The problem of reduction of brain weight in parkinsonism in relation to
physiological age atrophy is discussed. The decrease in brain and lenticular
nuclei weight in Huntington's disease corresponds well with the results of
previous quantitative and morphometric studies. The importance of absolute
values in the analysis of neurotransmitters and the need for standardized

quantitative dissection of particular brain areas for the understanding of the pathomechanisms of extrapyramidal disorders are emphasized.

Introduction

The measurement of certain neurotransmitter substances and their related biosynthetic enzymes in post-mortem brain tissue from patients dying with extrapyramidal disorders has provided a better understanding of the clinical features and the pathobiochemical basis of such conditions. However, there are considerable discrepancies in the results of such biochemical analyses reported by various laboratories (see *Bernheimer*, 1970; *Bowen et al.*, 1977; *Riederer* and *Wuketich*, 1976; *Winblad et al.*, 1978; *Mackay et al.*, 1978). Hence, the results published on particular loci of the brain may not be comparable with the results reported elsewhere. The standardized chemical analytical methods used are unlikely to be responsible for such deviations, but there are a number of variables to be considered, including: age, sex, cause of death, time of death, terminal hypoxia and agonal state, pre-mortem medication, brain weight, additional brain diseases, time elapsed between death and autopsy, storage time, and dissection technique (see *Bowen et al.*, 1977; *Bird* and *Iversen*, 1974; *Riederer* and *Wuketich*, 1976; *Mackay et al.*, 1978; *Winblad*, 1979). The need for uniform and standardized brain dissection techniques and definition of key areas, as well as the establishment of world-wide standards for the collection, processing, storage and disbursement of human nervous system specimens has been emphasized in the Human Brain Dissection Workshop sponsored by the NINCDS, held in Vienna in September 1979.

The purpose of this study, which is part of an investigation program on the regional distribution of biogenic amines within the human brain in physiological conditions and various diseases, is to present some results of quantitative dissection of some particular brain areas in controls and extrapyramidal disorders and the correlations between their fresh weights and biogenic amine values in controls and Parkinson's disease. Quantitative biochemical analysis was performed on the basis of quantitative dissection of five subcortical nuclei which are well delineated, easily recognized, and therefore can be totally removed.

Source Material

Whole brains were used from three groups of patients (Table 1).

Table 1. *Age, sex and death-autopsy intervals*

	Age	Sex M/F	Post-mortem interval (hours)
Controls (n = 17)	71.33 ± 0.26	9/8	7.9 ± 1.09
Parkinson's disease (n = 11)	76.5 ± 1.85	4/7	9.8 ± 2.4
Huntington's chorea (n = 4)	63.2 ± 1.9	2/2	8.2 ± 1.9

Means ± S.E.M. are indicated.

Controls

17 patients without history or findings suggestive of neurologic disorders who died of myocardial infarction (4 cases), pulmonary embolism (5 cases), acute heart failure (6 cases), rectal carcinoma and diabetes mellitus (one case each). None of them died in long-lasting coma and there were no brain injuries or encephalomalacias. The average age was 71.33 ± 0.26 years with a range of 65 to 80 years. Drug treatment included hemodiluting, dehydrating and heart drugs, antihypertensive agents, antibiotics and, in case of diabetes mellitus, insulin. The study excluded patients on medication that affects catecholamine metabolism (phenothiazines, Dopa, etc.). The time between death and necropsy averaged 7.9 ± 1.09 hours with a range from 3 to 12 hours.

Parkinson's Disease

11 patients with an average age of 76.5 ± 1.85 years (range 68—85 years) who had died of akinetic crisis, decubital sepsis or bronchopneumonia. Most of them had clinical evidence of mental symptoms including various degrees of dementia or confusional states. Drug treatment within one week before death included L-Dopa with a decarboxylase inhibitor and anticholinergic drugs. The post-mortem interval averaged 9.8 ± 2.3 hours with a range of 4 to 20 hours.

Huntington's Chorea

Four patients with a mean age of 63.2 ± 1.9 and an age range 57—67 years who had died of pneumonia and decubital sepsis.

The ante-mortem drug medication included neuroleptic drugs. The average post-mortem interval was 8.2 ± 1.9 hours with a range of 3 to 14 hours.

In all cases the cadaver reached the mortuary cold room (4 °C) within three hours of death and remained there until post-mortem examination was performed.

Dissection Methods

Once removed from the skull, the whole brain was weighed, then halved sagittaly. The right hemisphere was fixed in formalin for gross and histological examination; the left hemi-brain was immediately dissected in a cold room into a series of constituent areas. The following 5 areas were quantitatively dissected and totally removed: caudate nucleus, putamen, globus pallidus, nucleus amygdalae, and nucleus ruber. All brain areas were removed by the same examiner from a hemi-brain which had not been serially sliced according to a standardized preparation technique: The instruments used were a scalpel with a crescent shaped disposable blade and curbed scissors.

Caudate nucleus

In order to remove the caudate nucleus, the lateral ventricle is completely opened. The head and body of the caudate nucleus are removed medially from the deep hemispheral white matter and internal capsule by blunt dissection with a scalpel, and afterwards the whole nucleus including the tail is removed from the adjacent white matter using scissors. Once removed, the nucleus is cleaned from all adjacent portions of white matter, although small islands of white matter between the caudate nucleus and putamen may remain within the specimen. The head of the caudate nucleus is separated from the anterior part of the putamen by dividing the specimen in the middle of the head of the corpus striatum.

Putamen

Both the putamen and globus pallidus are prepared together. After dissection of the caudate nucleus coronal cuts of about 1 cm thickness are made through the basal ganglia, and these are found to demonstrate both parts of the lenticular nuclei. The putamen is excised from these coronal slices first using a scalpel, while the adjacent white matter of the internal and external capsules is removed with scissors. The only difficulty in the exact dissection of the putamen is caused by the gray matter extensions of the putamen into the internal capsule which are usually removed together with the white substance. The anterior commissure is also thoroughly removed from the base of the putamen.

Globus pallidus

This part of the lenticular nuclei is excised from the coronal slices through the basal ganglia, and the adjacent white substance of the internal capsule and the anterior commissure is removed with scissors. The internal and external parts of the pallidum are not separated.

Amygdala

A coronal section is taken through the entire body of the temporal lobe at the level just before the mammillary body and this is found to transect the anterior tip of the temporal horn of the lateral ventricle. The amygdala can then be shelled out from the anterior pole of the temporal lobe and is dissected with the scalpel from the adjacent cortex of the gyrus uncinatus and the hippocampal and parahippocampal gyri; the remaining gray and white matter surrounding the amygdala are thoroughly removed with scissors.

Nucleus ruber

A deep cut is made through the midbrain at the level of the superior colliculus in a plane at right angles to the long axis of the brainstem. The cut is made on the ventral surface of the brainstem just posterior to the mammillary body and emerging at the level of the upper border of the superior colliculi. It usually divides the nucleus ruber, of which the two round halves can be shelled out from the midbrain. The surrounding myelinated capsule and adjacent tissue are thoroughly removed with scissors.

Storage and Analysis

Once removed, each of the brain areas is weighed and then stored in sealed polyethylene plastic bags at —70 °C until analysis. The storage time of dissected material at —70 °C was 42 ± 5 days. Biochemical analyses were performed on freshly homogenized samples after reweighing. Aliquots from the same homogenate were used for dopamine, noradrenaline, and 5-HT estimations.

Dopamine was determined according to *Anton* and *Sayre* (1964); noradrenaline was assayed fluorometrically by the method of *Bertler et al.* (1958), and 5-HT was measured according to *Ashcroft* and *Sharman* (1962), modified by *Quay* (1963); calculations were made using internal standards.

Neuropathology

The right hemispheres were processed for neuropathology using routine histological techniques.

The control brains showed slight to moderate cortical neuronal loss and slight to moderate numbers of senile plaques and neurofibrillary tangles conforming to age. There were no cases of Pick's or Alzheimer's disease, and no considerable cerebrovascular or any other pathological lesions observed.

All cases of group 2 conformed to the standard histopathological criteria of Parkinson's disease without signs of postencephalitic parkinsonism or progressive supranuclear palsy. There was mild to moderate cortical atrophy with variable numbers of senile plaques and neurofibrillary tangles usually conforming to age.

The 4 cases of group 3 conformed to the standard criteria of Huntington's chorea with severe atrophy of the corpus striatum, and considerable cortical atrophy but without senile changes.

Results

Fresh Weight

The fresh weights of the whole brains and of the five completely removed brain areas were compared for the whole sample (Table 2). The average brain weight in the total group was 1163 ± 100.6 g; the fresh weight of the caudate nucleus was 5.34 ± 0.6 g, putamen 5.0 ± 0.8 g, globus pallidus 2.77 ± 0.50 g, nucleus ruber 1.18 ± 0.23 g, and amygdala 1.65 ± 0.41 g. Within the total groups there was a statistically significant correlation between the fresh weights of the whole brains and of the caudate nucleus, putamen, globus pallidus and amygdala, while no correlation was found between brain weight and the nucleus ruber.

Table 2. *Quantitative dissection of various human brain areas*

	Fresh weight [g]	Statistical correlation Whole brain/Brain areas	
		r	Sign.
Whole brain (n = 32)	1163 ± 100.6	—	—
Caudate n. (n = 32)	5.34± 0.62	0.5595	p < 0.01
Putamen (n = 32)	5.00± 0.80	0.5789	p < 0.01
Gl. pallidus (n = 32)	2.77± 0.5	0.4456	p < 0.02
N. ruber (n = 31)	1.18± 0.2	0.0721	n.s.
N. amygdalae (n = 30)	1.65± 0.41	0.3983	p < 0.05

Shown are means ± S.D. Number of brains in parenthesis.

Comparison of the mean fresh weights of the whole brains and of the various dissected brain areas was performed between the three groups.

In Huntington's chorea the mean whole brain weight (84.3 % of controls) and the average weight of the caudate nuclei (47.4 % of controls) and putamen (43.3 % of controls) were significantly lower than those in both the controls and the parkinsonian group, while this latter group did not considerably differ from controls

Table 3. *Quantitative dissection of human caudate nucleus in controls, parkinsonism, and Huntington's chorea*

	Fresh weight [g]	Statistical analysis
Controls		
Whole brain (n = 19)	1181.6 ± 154.8	r = 0.9020
Caudate n. (n = 19)	5.38 ± 0.56	p < 0.001
Parkinson's disease		
Whole brain (n = 13)	1136.2 ± 100.1[a]	r = 0.3866
Caudate n. (n = 13)	5.18 ± 0.63[a]	n.s.
Huntington's chorea		
Whole brain (n = 4)	995.0 ± 135.0[b]	
Caudate n. (n = 4)	2.55 ± 0.22[c]	

[a] n.s. = means ± S.D. not significantly different at p < 0.05 from respective control values.
[b] Different from controls p < 0.01.
[c] Different from controls p < 0.001.
Number of brains in parenthesis.

Table 4. *Correlation between the weight of whole brain and various brain areas in controls, parkinsonism, and Huntington's chorea*

Fresh weight [g]	Controls (19)		Parkinson's disease (13)		Huntington's chorea (4)		% decrease in chorea from controls
Whole brain	1181.6	± 154.8	1136.2	± 100.1	995.0	± 135.0	15.7[a]
Caudate n.	5.38 ±	0.56	5.18 ±	0.63	2.55 ±	0.22	52.6[b]
Putamen	4.99 ±	0.97	5.01 ±	0.57	2.16 ±	0.16	56.7[b]
Gl. pallidus	2.77 ±	0.5	2.76 ±	0.48	1.75 ±	0.11	36.8[b]
N. ruber	1.19 ±	0.23	1.16 ±	0.19	1.10 ±	0.12	0
N. amygdalae	1.65 ±	0.38	1.60 ±	0.42	1.68 ±	0.28	0

[a] Different from controls and parkinsonism p < 0.01.
[b] Different from controls and parkinsonism p < 0.001.
Number of brains in parenthesis.

Table 5. *Fresh weights and biogenic amine values in various brain areas in controls*

Brain region*	Fresh weight (g) (n = 19)	Dopamine (n = 15)		Noradrenaline (n = 10)		5-Hydroxytryptamine (n = 17)	
		nmol g^{-1}	nmol reg.$^{-1}$	nmol g^{-1}	nmol reg.$^{-1}$	nmol g^{-1}	nmol reg.$^{-1}$
Caudate n.	5.38 ± 0.56	24.18 ± 1.85	130 ± 9.75	0.57 ± 0.11	3.06 ± 0.23	1.65 ± 0.13	8.87 ± 0.65
Putamen	4.99 ± 0.97	25.82 ± 2.12	128.8 ± 0.85	0.27 ± 0.06	1.34 ± 0.09	1.45 ± 0.12	7.23 ± 0.60
Gl. pallidus	2.77 ± 0.50	5.16 ± 0.37	14.29 ± 1.10	0.24 ± 0.05	0.66 ± 0.05	2.15 ± 0.17	5.95 ± 0.36
N. amygdalae	1.65 ± 0.38	1.21 ± 0.09	2.0 ± 0.16	4.73 ± 0.83	7.81 ± 0.06	1.42 ± 0.09	2.32 ± 0.15
N. ruber	1.19 ± 0.23	5.2 ± 0.42	6.17 ± 0.53	1.43 ± 0.25	1.70 ± 0.05	3.37 ± 0.24	3.99 ± 0.27

* Total brain weight (n = 19) = 1181.6 ± 154.8 g.
All values are means ± S.D. Number of brains in parenthesis.
reg. = region

Table 6. *Fresh weights and biogenic amine values in various brain areas in Parkinson's disease*

Brain region	Fresh weight (g) (n = 13)	Dopamine (n = 18)		Noradrenaline (n = 15)		5-Hydroxytryptamine (n = 17)	
		nmol g^{-1}	nmol reg.$^{-1}$	nmol g^{-1}	nmol reg.$^{-1}$	nmol g^{-1}	nmol reg.$^{-1}$
Caudate n.	5.18 ± 0.63	2.48 ± 0.20	12.87 ± 1.10	0.26 ± 0.04	1.35 ± 0.09	0.71 ± 0.06	3.68 ± 0.27
Putamen	5.01 ± 0.57	1.28 ± 0.11	6.41 ± 0.45	0.15 ± 0.07	0.75 ± 0.05	0.80 ± 0.06	4.00 ± 0.30
Gl. pallidus	2.76 ± 0.48	0.65 ± 0.05	1.79 ± 0.14	0.19 ± 0.08	0.52 ± 0.04	0.74 ± 0.04	2.04 ± 0.15
N. amygdalae	1.60 ± 0.42	1.39 ± 0.10	2.23 ± 0.20	1.42 ± 0.19	2.27 ± 0.02	0.88 ± 0.07	1.41 ± 0.09
N. ruber	1.16 ± 0.19	0.59 ± 0.06	0.68 ± 0.06	0.47 ± 0.05	0.55 ± 0.04	2.16 ± 0.17	2.50 ± 0.22

Shown are means ± S.D. Number of brains in parenthesis.
reg. = region

(Tables 3, 4). The globus pallidus was less reduced in weight in Huntington's chorea (73.2 % of controls) and showed no definite weight reduction in parkinsonism, while the mean weights of the nucleus ruber and amygdala did not considerably differ between the three groups (Table 4).

Biogenic Amines

Comparison of fresh weights and of both the absolute and relative concentrations of DA, NE and 5-HT in the five dissected brain areas were performed for controls (Table 5) and Parkinson's disease (Table 6).

While in parkinsonian brains the fresh weights of the examined regions are not considerably reduced, there is a significant decrease of DA, NE and 5-HT in most areas. *DA reduction* is most pronounced in the basal ganglia; the putamen showing only 5 % of controls, caudate nucleus and globus pallidus 10 and 12 %, respectively, and nucleus ruber 11 % of controls. *NE values* are reduced in the following order of severity; amygdala (12 %), nucleus ruber (33 % of controls), caudate nucleus (45 % of controls), putamen (55 % of controls), and globus pallidus (80 % of controls). *5-HT values* in Parkinson's disease are reduced in globus pallidus (about 30 % of controls), caudate nucleus (44 % of controls), putamen (57 % of controls), and nucleus ruber and amygdala (64 and 62 % of controls, respectively).

Discussion

Quantitative dissection of some human brain areas has been performed in a series of autopsy cases with extrapyramidal disorders, *i.e.* Parkinson's disease and Huntington's chorea which were sex- and age-matched with controls who had died of cardiac failure and pulmonary embolism. Post-mortem time was similar in all three groups. There was a statistically significant correlation between the average fresh weights of the basal ganglia (caudate nucleus, putamen and globus pallidus) and of the whole brain which is in agreement with previous volumetric studies of the human brain (*Blinkov* and *Glezer*, 1968; *Orthner* and *Sendler*, 1968; *Kretschmann*, 1971), while *Schröder et al.* (1975) did not find any definite correlation between the volume of the corpus striatum and of the cerebral hemispheres. In our series of controls and of Parkinson's disease, the fresh weight of the caudate nucleus was slightly higher than that of the putamen, while according to most authors, the volume of the putamen is larger than that of the caudate nucleus (*Harman* and *Carpenter*, 1950;

Hopf, 1965; *Jungklaass* and *Orthner*, 1960; *Kretschmann*, 1971; *Schröder et al.*, 1975), the differences ranging from 2 % (*Kretschmann*, 1971) to 27 % (*Harman* and *Carpenter*, 1958). These differences may at least in part result from local variations in the fluid content which in caudate nucleus has been found to be higher than in the putamen (*Riederer* and *Wuketich*, 1976). For smaller brain areas, *i.e.* nucleus ruber and amygdala, no such correlations with total brain weight were found which may reflect some difficulties in the exact quantitative dissection of such small brain loci as demonstrated by the comparatively high standard deviations of their weights (Tables 3 and 4).

The weights of the lenticular nuclei in our controls are within the wide range of divergent data reported by various authors, the weight of the caudate nucleus in adult man ranging from about 13 g (*Blinkov* and *Glezer*, 1968) to 3.5 g (*Bowen*, pers. communic.) and 2.5 g (*Bird* and *Iversen*, 1974).

No significant differences in the average weights of the whole brain and subcortical nuclei were found between the group of parkinsonian patients and age-matched controls. Our data indicating normal weight of the globus pallidus are in accordance with *Sabuncu* (1969) who found no morphometric differences in this nucleus between parkinsonian patients and controls. The average fresh weight of parkinsonian brains in this series was comparable with that of 100 histologically verified cases of Parkinson's disease, many of them with dementia or mental disturbances. Their age averaged 71.8 ± 0.92 years (range 52 to 86 years) and the duration of illness 8.61 ± 0.76 years (1—27 years). In this latter group the average brain weight was 1151 ± 20.1 g with a range from 910 to 1400 g (*Grisold et al.*, unpubl.). Our data differ from those reported by *Hakim* and *Mathieson* (1979) indicating that the average brain weight in demented parkinsonian patients (1281 ± 21.8 g) was significantly less than the average for non-demented age-matched controls (1365 ± 25.1 g) at the 0.02 level. Although no psychometric data were available for our controls, the average brain weight in this series was in the lower border line values of those reported for non-demented persons between 70 and 79 years of age (*Bürger*, 1960; *Tomlinson et al.*, 1968; *Haug*, 1975; *Corsellis*, 1976).

Brain atrophy has been documented by CT in both Parkinson's disease (*Becker et al.*, 1979; *Schneider et al.*, 1979) and physiological and pathological aging (*Huckman et al.*, 1975; *Barron et al.*, 1976; *Haug*, 1977; *Earnest et al.*, 1979; *Meese et al.*, 1979). Brain atrophy in Parkinson's disease has been found to be related to age, sex and duration of the disease (*Becker et al.*, 1979). Although comparison of CT ventricular measurements appear to confirm the assumption deduced from previous PEG studies (*Selby*, 1968) that brain atrophy in parkinsonian patients is more prevalent than in normal patients within the scope of age involution, there is as yet no definite proof that brain atrophy in Parkinson's disease exceeds the physiological age atrophy of the brain (*Becker et al.*, 1979).

Conversely, in Huntington's chorea, the average weights of both the whole brain and the lenticular nuclei were significantly lower than those in controls and parkinsonian patients which confirms earlier reports (*Bruyn*, 1968; *Bird* and *Iversen*, 1974). The weight reduction of the caudate nucleus and putamen which in our series was 52.6 and 56.7 %, respectively as compared to 49 and 54 %, respectively, in *Bird* and *Iversen*'s (1974) choreic series is much higher than that of the whole brain (84.3 and 85 % of controls, respectively). The globus pallidus was less reduced in weight—36.8 % of controls in our series and 37 % in the series of *Bird* and *Iversen* (1974), while no weight reduction was found for the nucleus ruber and amygdala. The weight decrease of the basal ganglia in Huntington's chorea is also comparable with the results of quantitative and morphometric studies in serial brain sections by *Lange et al.* (1976) who reported an average volume reduction of 56 % for the striatum, 58 % for the lateral pallidum and 50 % for the medial pallidum, while reduction of both the average fresh brain weight and fresh volume of the cerebral hemispheres in choreic brains were about 20 % of the controls as compared to 12.7 % in our series. Volume loss of the neostriatum in Huntington's chorea is due to depletion of the medium and small neurons reaching 70 to 80 %, and glial cell loss amounting to 25 % (*Lange et al.*, 1976; *Bruyn et al.*, 1979).

Another point to be discussed is the fact that concentrations of chemical substances are usually given in gram/wet weight. Since different regions of the brain show slight variations in specific weight (*Blinkov* and *Glezer*, 1968) and in water content (*Riederer* and *Wuketich*, 1976) which might be influenced by long-term freezing storage, it may be more accurate to relate concentrations to g/dry weight or protein content. However, due to the limitations of available tissue these types of calculation are rarely used.

All three types of calculations, however, neglect the absolute value of a substance per weight of brain areas. It appears of interest, therefore, that the loss of dopamine in the striatum of parkinsonian patients is almost the same as the decrease of homovanillic acid (HVA) in the cerebrospinal fluid (CSF) of patients with Parkinson's disease (*Curzon et al.*, 1970; *Papeschi et al.*, 1972; *Rinne et al.*, 1973; *Sourkes*, 1975). Since about 75 % of the DA in the mammalian brain is present in the nigrostriatal system, the level of HVA measured in lumbar CSF is believed largely to reflect the functional activity of this pathway. How a certain brain area contributes to the changes of neurotransmitters measurable in the CSF depends not only on the concentration of a given substance per gram tissue or the degree of innervation, but also on the size of the particular brain area. Tables 5 and 6 demonstrate the correlations of DA, NE and 5-HT contents given both in relative concentrations per gram brain tissue and in absolute values related to the total weight of the respective brain loci. In Parkinson's disease almost normal weights of the subcortical nuclei are associated with significant loss of DA particularly in the putamen, caudate nucleus and globus pallidus with slight to moderate decrease of NE and 5-HT in these nuclei, while nucleus ruber and amygdala demonstrate variable changes of these monoamines. Since Parkinson's disease does not become clinically manifest before the loss of striatal dopamine reaches 75 to 80 % of its normal values (*Carlsson*, 1974; *Riederer* and *Wuketich*, 1976), the striatum is considered to have a compensatory mechanism preventing the occurrence of parkinsonian symptoms over a long life span. This mechanism may in part be reflected by the storage capacity of the total striatal region. Therefore, quantitative dissection is important in obtaining average values of particular biochemical parameters in a brain region. However, a correlation of subregional histopathological disturbances with biochemical changes in the same sample may well provide a better understanding of the underlying pathomechanisms of extrapyramidal and related disorders. The lack of information on the fine anatomical structure of these brain areas is a further difficulty requiring examination. Consideration of absolute amounts of neurotransmitter substances in certain brain loci may therefore provide a better understanding of the neurochemical basis of some extrapyramidal disorders.

References

Anton, A. H., Sayre, D. F.: The distribution of dopamine and Dopa in various animals and a method for their determination in diverse biological material. J. Pharmacol. Exp. Ther. *145*, 326—336 (1964).

Ashcroft, G. W., Sharman, D. F.: Drug induced changes in the concentration of 5-OR indolyl compounds in the cerebrospinal fluid and caudate nucleus. Brit. J. Pharmacol. *19*, 153—160 (1962).

Barron, S. A., Jacobs, L., Kinkel, W. R.: Changes in size of normal lateral ventricles during aging determined by computerized tomography. Neurology (Minneap.) *26*, 1011—1013 (1976).

Becker, H., Schneider, E., Hacker, H., Fischer, P. A.: Cerebral atrophy in Parkinson's disease—represented in CT. Arch. Psychiat. Nervenkr. *227,* 81—88 (1979).

Bernheimer, H.: Biochemical parameters of catecholamine and 5-hydroxy-tryptamine metabolism with particular regard human brain. In: Neuropathology: Methods and Diagnosis (*Tedeschi, G.,* ed.), pp. 797—823. New York: Little, Brown & Co. 1970.

Bertler, A., Carlsson, A., Rosengren, E.: A method for the fluorometric determination of adrenaline and noradrenaline in tissues. Acta Physiol. Scand. *44,* 273—292 (1958).

Bird, E. D., Iversen, L. L.: Huntington's chorea. Post-mortem measurement of glutamic acid decarboxylase, choline acetyltransferase and dopamine in basal ganglia. Brain *97,* 457—472 (1974).

Blinkov, S. M., Glezer, I. I.: Das Zentralnervensystem in Zahlen und Tabellen. Jena: VEB Fischer. 1968.

Bowen, D. B., Smith, C. B., White, P., Goodhardt, M. J., Spillane, J. A., Flack, R. H., Davison, A. N.: Chemical pathology of the organic dementias. I. Validity of biochemical measurements on human post-mortem brain specimens. Brain *100,* 397—426 (1977).

Bruyn, G. W.: Huntington's disease. In: Handbook of Clinical Neurology (*Vinken, P. J., Bruyn, G. W.,* eds.), Vol. 6, pp. 298—378. Amsterdam: North-Holland. 1968.

Bruyn, G. W., Bots, G. Th. A. M., Dom, R.: Huntington's chorea: current neuropathological status. In: Advances in Neurology, Vol. 23 (*Chase, T. N., et al.,* eds.), pp. 83—93. New York: Raven Press. 1979.

Bürger, M.: Altern und Krankheit als Problem der Biomorphose. Leipzig: Thieme. 1960.

Carlsson, A.: The "on-off" effect. In: Advances in Neurology (*McDowell, F., Barbeau, A.,* eds.), Vol. 5, pp. 367—368. New York: Raven Press. 1974.

Corsellis, J. A. N.: Ageing and the dementias. In: Greenfield's Neuropathology (*Blackwood, W., Corsellis, J. A. N.,* eds.), 3rd ed., pp. 796—848. London: E. Arnold. 1976.

Curzon, G., Godwin-Austen, R. B., Tomlinson, E. B., Kantamaneni, B. D.: The cerebrospinal fluid homovanillic acid concentrations in patients with parkinsonism treated with L-dopa. J. Neurol. Neurosurg. Psychiat. *33,* 1—6 (1970).

Earnest, M. P., Heaton, R. K., Wilkinson, W. E., Manke, W. F.: Cortical atrophy, ventricular enlargement and intellectual impairment in the aged. Neurology (Minneap.) *29,* 1138—1143 (1979).

Grisold, W., Jellinger, K., Danielczyk, W.: Brain atrophy in Parkinson's disease. (In preparation.)

Hakim, A. M., Mathieson, G.: Dementia in Parkinson disease: a neuropathologic study. Neurology (Minneap.) *29,* 1209—1214 (1979).

Harman, P. J., Carpenter, M. B.: Volumetric comparisons of the basal ganglia of various mammalia including man. J. comp. Neurol. *93,* 125—137 (1958).

Haug, G.: Age and sex dependence of the size of normal ventricles on computed tomography. Neuroradiol. *14*, 201—204 (1977).

Haug, H.: Neuere Aspekte über den biologischen Alterungsvorgang im menschlichen Gehirn. Verh. Anat. Ges. *69*, 380—395 (1975).

Huckman, M. S., Fox, J., Topel, J.: The validity of criteria for the evaluation of cerebral atrophy by computed tomography. Radiology *116*, 85—92 (1975).

Jungklaass, F. K., Orthner, H.: Über quantitative Beziehungen im Stammhirn. Dtsch. Z. Nervenkr. *181*, 62—70 (1960).

Kretschmann, H. J.: Biometrische Untersuchungen der Frischvolumina menschlicher Hirnregionen. Verh. Anat. Ges. *65*, 139—145 (1971).

Lange, H., Thörner, G., Hopf, A., Schröder, F. K.: Morphometric studies of the neuropathological changes in choreatic diseases. J. neurol. Sci. *28*, 401—425 (1976).

Mackay, A. V. P., Davies, P., Dewar, A. J., Yates, C. M.: Regional distribution of enzymes associated with neurotransmission by monoamines, acetylcholine and GABA in the human brain. J. Neurochem. *30*, 827 to 839 (1978).

Meese, W., Kluge, W., Grumme, T., Hopfenmüller, W.: Der normale Liquorraum im Computer-Tomogramm. J. Neurol. (in press).

Orthner, H., Sendler, W.: Einige Ergebnisse makroskopisch-quantitativer Hirnforschung. Verh. Dtsch. Ges. Path. *52*, 243—253 (1968).

Papeschi, R., Molina-Negro, P., Sourkes, T. L., Erba, G.: The concentration of homovanillic and 5-hydroxyindoleacetic acids in ventricular and lumbar CSF. Neurol. (Minneap.) *22*, 1151—1159 (1972).

Quay, W. B.: Differential extractions for the spectrofluorometric measurement of diverse 5-hydroxy- and 5-methoxyindoles. Anal. Biochem. *5*, 51—59 (1963).

Riederer, P., Wuketich, St.: Time course of nigrostriatal degeneration in Parkinson's disease. J. Neural Transm. *38*, 277—301 (1976).

Rinne, U. K., Sonninen, V., Siirtola, T.: Acid monoamine metabolites in the cerebrospinal fluid of parkinsonian patients treated with levodopa alone or combined with a decarboxylase inhibitor. Europ. Neurol. *9*, 349—356 (1973).

Sabuncu, N.: Quantitative Untersuchungen am Pallidum beim Parkinsonsyndrom. Dtsch. Z. Nervenheilk. *196*, 40—48 (1969).

Selby, G.: Brain atrophy in parkinsonism. J. neurol. Sci. *6*, 517—559 (1968).

Schneider, E., Fischer, P. A., Jacobi, P., Becker, H., Hacker, H.: The significance of cerebral atrophy for the symptomatology of Parkinson's disease. J. neurol. Sci. *42*, 187—197 (1979).

Schröder, K. F., Hopf, A., Lange, H., Thörner, G.: Morphometrisch-statistische Strukturanalysen des Striatum, Pallidum und Nucleus subthalamicus beim Menschen. I. Striatum. J. Hirnforsch. *16*, 333—350 (1975).

Sourkes, T. L.: On the origin of homovanillic acid (HVA) in the cerebrospinal fluid. J. Neural Transm. *34*, 153—157 (1975).

Tomlinson, B. E., Blessed, G., Roth, M.: Observations on the brains of non-demented old people. J. neurol. Sci. *7,* 331—356 (1968).

Winblad, B.: Post-mortem dissection of human brain. Paper presented at Human Brain Dissection Workshop, Vienna, September 14—15, 1979.

Authors' address: Doz. Dr. *P. Riederer,* Ludwig Boltzmann-Institute of Clinical Neurobiology, Lainz-Hospital, Wolkersbergenstrasse 1, A-1130 Wien, Austria.

Journal of Neural Transmission, Suppl. 16, 69—81 (1980)
© by Springer-Verlag 1980

On the Mechanism of the Antiparkinsonian Action of 1-DOPA and Bromocriptine: A Theoretical and Experimental Analysis of Dopamine Receptor Sub- and Supersensitivity

L. F. Agnati and K. Fuxe

Department of Human Physiology, University of Bologna, Bologna, Italy, and
Department of Histology, Karolinska Institutet, Stockholm, Sweden

With 6 Figures

Summary

Further advancements in the development of antiparkinsonian drugs are highly dependent on a better understanding of the biochemical changes present in the "supersensitive DA receptors". The present paper stresses also the importance of the development of behavioural models for studies on supersensitive DA receptors (rotational behaviour in 6-OHDA lesioned rats) and on intact DA receptors, *i.e.* rotational behaviour in KA lesioned rats. The relevance of heuristic models for DA receptor sub- and super-sensitivity is underlined. The pharmacological findings with bromocriptine indicate that its ability to reduce the on-off phenomenon in patients could be due to its longlasting and rather constant activation of supersensitive DA receptors, and its partial DA agonist activity at DA receptors not linked to adenylate cyclase. The concept is introduced that to understand DA receptor sub-supersensitivity it is of help to postulate variations in the numbers of coupled DA receptors as an important factor. The behavioural experiments with elymoclavine further underline this view by indicating increases in the working range at supersensitive DA receptors although the amount of agonist is reduced.

Furthermore, the concept has been introduced that the DA receptor supersensitivity development does not depend only on the deficit of the transmitter but possibly also on the deficit of a presynaptically released trophic factor. This factor could play a critical role in the control of the biochemical machinery of the postsynaptic cell, *e.g.* receptor synthesis, formation of catalytic units and of compounds which can enhance the coupling between receptors and the biological effector.

The introduction of l-DOPA in the treatment of Parkinson's disease was a major break-through in neurology (*Birkmayer* and *Hornykiewicz*, 1962; *Cotzias et al.*, 1967). The l-DOPA therapy could be further improved by combining the l-DOPA treatment with a peripheral decarboxylase inhibitor (see e.g. *Birkmayer et al.*, 1974; *Rinne*, 1978). With the combined treatment it became possible to avoid peripheral side-effects of DOPA treatment since peripheral formation of dopamine (DA) was blocked. In this way only a central accumulation of DA could occur. However, in recent studies it has been noticed that following a 5—7-year treatment with l-DOPA, the original marked improvement of rigidity, hypokinesia and tremor was reduced or disappeared in a substantial number of parkinsonian patients (see *Ludin* and *Bass-Verrey*, 1976; *Marsden* and *Parkes*, 1976, 1977; *Hornykiewicz*, 1974; *Rinne*, 1978). Furthermore, half of the patients on long-term treatment with l-DOPA develops on-off phenomena. This phenomenon means that the patient has an on-period characterized by marked hyperkinesias followed by an off-period characterized by marked hypokinesia. The off-period can last for a variable number of hours. Against this background it has been of substantial interest to observe that the dopamine receptor agonist, bromocriptine (CB 154), seems capable of reducing the number of patients exhibiting on-off phenomena on l-DOPA treatment. Furthermore, bromocriptine produces a further improvement of the motor functions in parkinsonian patients, further reducing rigidity, hypokinesia and tremor (see *Calne et al.*, 1974, 1978; *Lieberman et al.*, 1976, 1979; *Marsden* and *Parkes*, 1976, 1977; *Parkes et al.*, 1976).

In the present paper we have tried to increase the understanding of these clinical results by studying the pharmacology of l-DOPA, bromocriptine (*Hökfelt* and *Fuxe*, 1972; *Fuxe*, 1973; *Fuxe et al.*, 1974; *Corrodi et al.*, 1973; *Johnsson et al.*, 1976) and elymoclavine (see *Fuxe et al.*, 1978 a) and by considering some theoretical aspects on DA receptor sub- and supersensitivity.

Pharmacological Studies on Bromocriptine

The available pharmacological evidence indicates that bromocriptine is a mixed dopamine receptor agonist-antagonist which only can activate one type of DA receptor, that is the type which is not linked to DA sensitive adenylate cyclase (*Markstein et al.*, 1978; *Fuxe et al.*, 1978 a, b; *Spano et al.*, 1976). Bromocriptine has affinity not only for agonist binding sites as studied with the radioligands ^{3}H-dopamine, ^{3}H-apomorphine and ^{3}H-ADTN (*Goldstein et al.*,

1978; *Fuxe et al.*, 1979 a) but also for antagonist binding sites of the DA receptors using radioligands such as ^{3}H-haloperidol and ^{3}H-spiperone (*Burt et al.*, 1978 a, b; *Fuxe et al.*, 1978 b; *Goldstein et al.*, 1978). Bromocriptine can probably act at DA receptors located both on axon terminals belonging to cortical striatal fibres and on cell bodies and their dendrites in the neostriatum.

As seen in Fig. 1, bromocriptine like l-DOPA and apomorphine can produce an activation of supersensitive DA receptors as shown by the induction of marked contralateral rotational behaviour in animals with a unilateral 6-hydroxydopamine induced lesion of the ascending DA pathways (*Ungerstedt* and *Arbuthnott*, 1970). In Fig. 1, the doses used are three times threshold doses, and it is clear

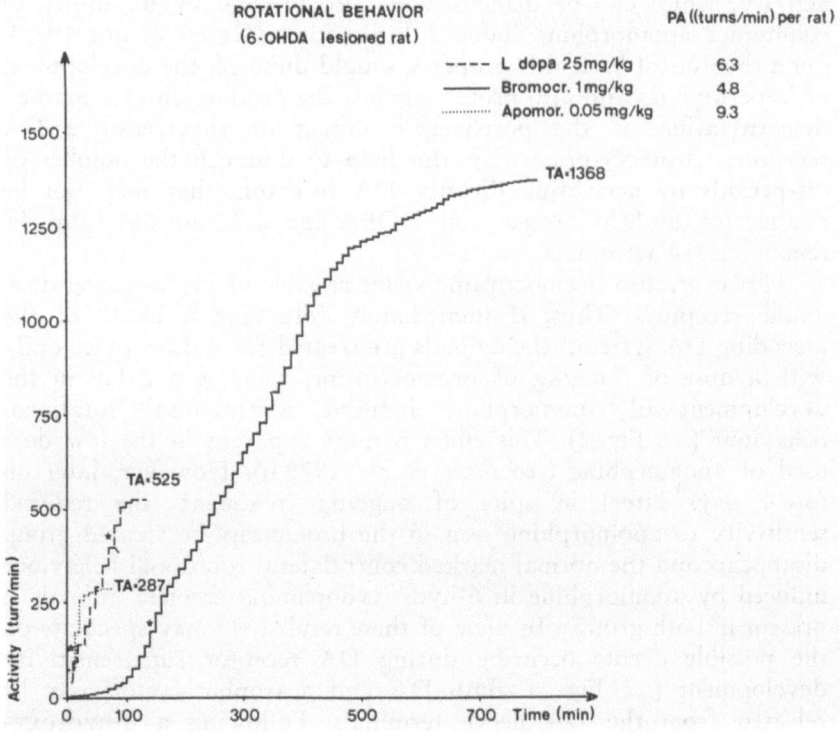

Fig. 1. The effects of l-DOPA, apomorphine and bromocriptine on rotational behaviour in rats with a unilateral 6-hydroxydopamine induced lesion of the ascending dopamine pathways. The animals (n = 4) were operated upon 3 to 4 months before testing of the drugs. The contralateral rotational behaviour induced by these three dopaminergic drugs in the doses (i.p.) shown in the figure is given on the Y-axis by showing the accumulation of turns per rat with time. The peak activity is indicated with an asterisk. All the injected doses represent three times a threshold dose

that bromocriptine unlike l-DOPA and apomorphine produces a rotational behaviour of long duration which is maintained at a rather constant rate over several hours. In monkeys with ventromedial tegmental lesions, bromocriptine also produces a prolonged relief of tremor (*Miyamoto et al.*, 1974). It therefore seems likely that part of the explanation for the ability of bromocriptine to diminish the on-off phenomenon in Parkinsonian patients on l-DOPA treatment can be due to its ability to produce a prolonged and constant activation of supersensitive DA receptors. Such a prolonged activation cannot be produced by l-DOPA even in the presence of peripheral decarboxylase inhibition. Another factor to consider is, however, as pointed out above, that bromocriptine also possesses antagonist activity, which can be demonstrated also *in vivo* by its ability to counteract apomorphine induced locomotion (Ögren *et al.*, 1979). On a theoretical basis this property should diminish the development of hyperkinesias and also protect against the production of a marked desensitization of the postsynaptic intact or supersensitive DA receptors. Bromocriptine may also help to diminish the number of off-periods by activating directly DA receptors that may not be reached by the DA formed from DOPA and diffusing out from the remaining DA terminals.

However, also bromocriptine seems capable of desensitizing dopamine receptors. Thus, if immediately following a lesion of the ascending DA systems, the animals are treated for 4 days twice daily with a dose of 5 mg/kg of bromocriptine, there is a delay in the development of apomorphine induced contralateral rotational behaviour (see Fig. 2). This effect is most apparent in the low dose used of apomorphine (see *Fuxe et al.*, 1979 b). However, later on (3—4 days later) in spite of ongoing treatment, the reduced sensitivity to apomorphine seen in the bromocriptine treated group disappears and the normal marked contralateral rotational behaviour induced by apomorphine in 6-hydroxydopamine lesioned animals is present in both groups. In view of these results, we may speculate on the possible events occuring during DA receptor supersensitivity development (see Fig. 3). Both DA and a trophic factor may be released from the DA nerve terminals. Following a 6-hydroxydopamine induced lesion of the DA pathway a supersensitivity phenomenon starts to develop in the DA receptor complex and in the intracellular biochemical machinery which may be controlled by the trophic factor. It seems as if bromocriptine initially can prevent the gradual increase of the biological response with time, which develops as a result of a DA deficit at the DA receptors. However, it cannot prevent the development of "delayed" supersensitivity. By this term

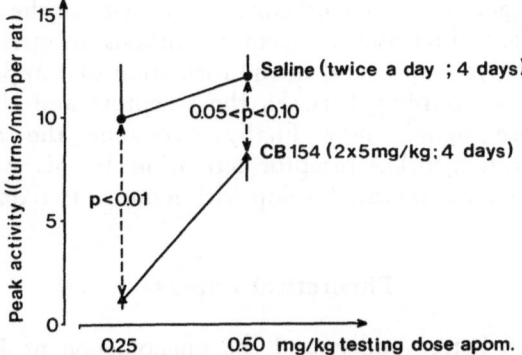

Fig. 2. The effects of chronic bromocriptine treatment on the apomorphine induced contralateral rotational behaviour in rats with a 6-OHDA induced lesion of the ascending DA pathways on one side of the brain. 6-OHDA was injected into the substantia nigra as described by *Ungerstedt* and *Arbuthnott* (1970). In relation to the 6-OHDA injection half of the animals (8 rats) were injected with bromocriptine (CB 154) in a dose of 10 mg/kg, while the other half of the animals (8 rats) received solvent treatment. Bromocriptine was given twice daily in a dose of 5 mg/kg for four days and the animals were tested for apomorphine induced rotational behaviour in the morning of the fifth day, the last injection of bromocriptine having been made in the afternoon of the previous day. Two i.p. doses of apomorphine were tested as indicated in the figure. On the Y-axis the peak activities are shown. Peak activities are given as means ± S.E.M. Statistical analysis was made by means of Mann-Whitney U-test. Note the reduction of apomorphine induced rotational behaviour in the bromocriptine group especially following treatment with 0.25 mg/kg of apomorphine

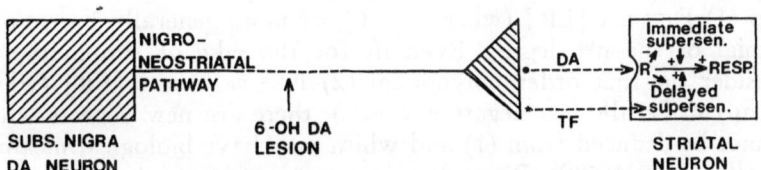

Fig. 3. A schematic illustration of possible events occuring at dopamine receptor sites during supersensitivity development. It is postulated that following a lesion of the nigrostriatal dopamine pathway there is a reduction of release not only of dopamine, the neurotransmitter, but also of a trophic factor controlling the biochemical machinery of the striatal nerve cells. The biological effector mechanism is controlled by the dopamine receptor activity and by biochemical processes in the nerve cell membrane such as receptor synthesis, synthesis of coupling proteins etc. These latter processes may mainly be under the control of a trophic factor released from the dopamine nerve terminals. Treatment with bromocriptine can initially delay the development of degeneration induced dopamine receptor supersensitivity. However, after a time period of about 5—8 days the so-called delayed supersensitivity development due to the lack of release of the trophic factor overcomes the inhibitory influence of the desensitizing process induced by the dopamine receptor stimulation and the response to the agonist is markedly enhanced

we mean a triggering of the biochemical machinery in the postsynaptic cell leading *e.g.* to increases in receptor synthesis, in increased formation of the catalytic units and in the formation of compounds which can enhance the coupling between the receptors and the biological effector. These signals may finally overcome the desensitizing influence of prolonged DA receptor activation. In this way a marked supersensitivity reaction can develop within one or two days.

Theoretical Aspects

In order to better understand the phenomenon of DA receptor sub- and supersensitivity and the development of on-off phenomena in Parkinsonian patients on l-DOPA treatment we would like to discuss the deductions which can be made from the possible existence of a threshold occupancy, a working range and a spare receptor fraction of DA receptors. The speculations, which can be made, may be helpful in the understanding of sub- and supersensitivity phenomena at DA receptor sites in the central nervous system. We would like to introduce the following theoretical base for such a concept.

Let us now consider some aspects of ligand (L) receptor (R) interaction as they appear from a comparison of radioligand evaluation and pharmacological studies. The occupancy theory states that the response (E) is related to the receptor occupation by the relationship (1) $E = a \times [LR]$ (where $a > 0$), or more generally by a polynomial of the nth degree. Even if, for the sake of simplicity, we consider the first order polynomial (2) $E = a_0 + a_1 \times [LR]$ (where a_0, a_1 can be allowed negative values), there are new aspects which cannot be deduced from (1) and which may have biological meaning (*Hollenberg*, 1978). Precisely, one can envisage that a certain threshold signal must be generated, that is a minimal fraction of the available receptors must be occupied, before a biological response can be observed:

$$f_T = \frac{[LR]_T}{[R_t]} > 0,$$ thus f_T is the minimum fraction of receptors which has to be occupied before a response can be observed. Furthermore, one can also envisage that the occupancy of a fraction of the available receptors is sufficient to trigger the maximal biological response:

$$f_M = \frac{[LR]_M}{[R_t]} < 1,$$ thus f_M is the fraction of receptors occupied when the response is maximal. Obviously it is always true $f_M > f_T$.

Thus, from equation (2.) and equation $K_D = \dfrac{[L]\,([R_t] - [LR])}{[LR]}$

it can be derived (see 5) (3.) $[L_t] = \dfrac{K_D\,[F\,(f_M - f_T) + f_T]}{1 - [F\,(f_M - f_T) + f_T]} +$

$[F\,(f_M - f_T) + f_T]\,[R_t]$.

Where $[L_t]$ is the ligand total concentration, F is the fractional response observed (*i.e.* $F = E/E_{mx}$), and $[R_t]$ is the receptor total concentration. Since in many cases $[R_t] \ll K_D$, then when $F = 0.5$ (half-maximal response is observed), equation (3.) gives

(4.) $[L_t]\,0.5 = ED_{50} = K_D \dfrac{f_M + f_T}{2 - (f_M + f_T)}$

Thus, only when $(f_M + f_T) = 1$ the $[L_t]\,0.5$ value (*i.e.* the ED_{50} value) is equal to the value of the true K_D. It is possible to illustrate these concepts by plots as those of Fig. 4 A and 4 B.—In fact, in Fig. 4 A the three receptor fractions (*i.e.* the "threshold receptor" fraction) $f_M - f_T$ (*i.e.* the "working range" fraction) and $1 - f_M$ (*i.e.* the "spare receptor" fraction) are shown. In Fig. 4 B the particular condition $f_M = 1 - f_T$ is shown under which $ED_{50} = K_D$.

The conclusions that can be reached are highly relevant. Thus, if one can prove that when $f = 0.5$ also $F = 0.5$, then in the frame of a situation like that just described one can assess not only that $ED_{50} = K_D$ but also that any possible threshold occupancy fraction is equal to the spare receptor fraction, and also the vice versa holds. Thus, it would be enough to find out that in a certain situation under study the f_T value is equal to the spare receptor fraction to be able to use the relationship $ED_{50} = K_D$. On the contrary (and this is certainly more common) it will be enough to find out that there exists a threshold fraction of receptor occupancy but not a spare receptor fraction (or vice versa) to conclude that $ED_{50} \neq K_D$. From a more general point of view we think that the existence, at least for some classes of receptors of a "threshold occupancy" fraction; a "working range" fraction; a "spare receptor" fraction, as stated above may allow some speculations to understand phenomena of receptor regulation in CNS.

In fact, the present theoretical considerations illustrate well the possibility that postsynaptic biological effector mechanisms can be regulated by processes controlling the number of receptors present in the working range. It seems possible that at least one of the mechanisms for the development of supersensitivity at postsynaptic DA receptors in the brain, is an increase in the working range of the DA receptors (coupled receptors) which is associated with the reduction in the number of spare receptors and in the fraction of receptors

necessary to induce a threshold response. This could represent one of
the mechanisms for the development of involuntary movements in
Parkinsonian patients treated with 1-DOPA, the so-called hyperkinesias. The biological effector unit of the DA receptor complex may
become frequently activated due to the very low fraction of dopamine receptors needed to induce a biological response in the nerve
cell membrane, leading to a change in ion permeability and thus in the
electrical characteristics of the membrane. The behavioural correlate
of such events may be the appearance of the involuntary movements.
In addition, the reduction in the number of spare receptors could be
one of the factors responsible for the development of supramaximal

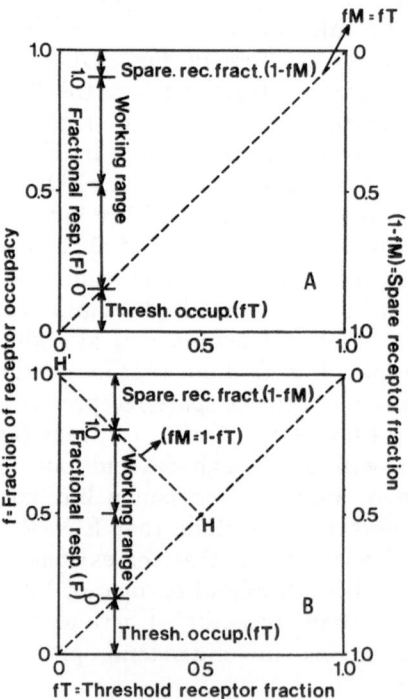

Fig. 4. *A.* Schematic representation of receptor occupation. It is important to
underline that by fixing the f_T value (threshold occupancy fraction) only the lower
limit of the "working range" (*i.e.* the range of receptor occupancy [f] in which
one can observe with an increase in f values an increase in the fractional response)
is determined. The upper limit can be determined either by knowing the f_M value
(fraction of receptor occupancy for the maximal response), or the spare receptor
fraction present ($= 1 - f_M$). *B.* As long as f_M assumes any value of the interval
HH′, the true K_D value can be obtained from the ED_{50}. It is important to underline
that, in this condition, by fixing the f_T value not only the lower but also the upper
limit of the working range is determined

biological responses. Hyperkinesias could represent such a supra-maximal response. One purpose for the threshold fraction of receptors may be to prevent synaptic noise to induce biological responses while the fraction of spare receptors may prevent an overactivation of biological effectors by binding the DA released without coupling it to an effector mechanism. A similar mechanism at the dopamine receptor sites may also be responsible for the development of tardive dyskinesias (*Baldessarini*, 1979) following long-term treatment with neuroleptics in schizophrenic patients. It seems possible that *e.g.* a combined increase of synthesis of coupling proteins and of receptor units, could produce the increase in the fraction of receptors coupled to the biological signal. These theoretical considerations may also explain why in several studies only small increases in the number of binding sites have been observed at DA receptor sites which probably are supersensitive. The important change may instead be in the number of coupled dopamine receptors.

When discussing this last point the following behavioural observations should also be considered. Rotational behaviour can be induced in animals by DA receptor agonists at both intact DA receptor sites and at supersensitive DA receptor sites. When using 6-hydroxy-dopamine induced lesions of the DA pathways the rotational behaviour is controlled by the supersensitive DA receptors. When instead a unilateral lesion of the striatum is induced by means of a neurotoxin, such as kainic acid which produces a degeneration of the striatal nerve cells, the elymoclavine induced rotational behaviour is instead controlled and induced by activation of intact DA receptors located on the unlesioned side (*Schwarcz et al.*, 1979).

The dose effect curves with elymoclavine are now compared in these two groups of rats. It is apparent that although the dose range of elymoclavine is considerably less in absolute amounts in the animals with supersensitive DA receptors the range of the biological response is much greater in this group of animals. The results show that, although there are less molecules of elymoclavine, the range for the biological signal is increased in rats having supersensitive DA receptors. These results support the above speculation and it should perhaps also be considered that not only may there be an increase in the number of coupled DA receptors but also in the number of catalytic units which are linked to each DA receptor complex (Fig. 6). Such mechanisms could elegantly explain also the increase in the slope values found in the dose effect curve in rats with super-sensitive DA receptors (*Schwarcz et al.*, 1979).

Subsensitivity development of postsynaptic receptor mechanisms could be related to an increase in the fraction of the receptors needed

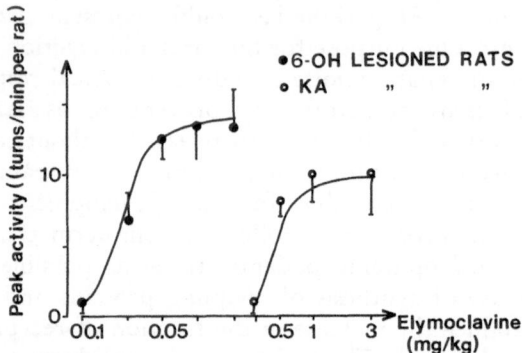

Fig. 5. Comparisons of the effects of elymoclavine on rotational behaviour produced in 6-hydroxydopamine lesioned or kainic acid lesioned animals. The 6-hydroxydopamine induced lesion was made in the substantia nigra three months before testing. This model results in development of dopamine receptor super-sensitivity in the striatum of the lesioned side and elymoclavine will produce contralateral rotational behaviour. In the kainic acid model the lesion is produced in the striatum as such by means of intrastriatal injections of kainic acid (0.5 μg per 1 μl). This injection will produce a marked disappearance of nerve cells within the striatum without producing degeneration of extrinsic terminals, such as the dopamine nerve terminals. In these animals the rotational behaviour induced by elymoclavine has an ipsilateral direction and is induced via activation of intact dopamine receptors located on the unoperated contralateral side. The dose effect curves are shown. Means ± S.E.M. (n = 4). The results show that the super-sensitive dopamine receptors react to much lower doses of elymoclavine and that the working range of the supersensitive dopamine receptors is increased compared to that of the intact dopamine receptors. Note that the maximal action of elymoclavine at supersensitive dopamine receptors is reached at a dose which is lower than the threshold dose found in the experiments with the kainic acid lesioned rats

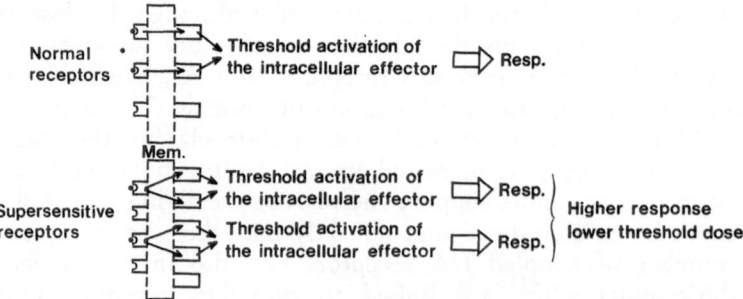

Fig. 6. Schematic illustration of possible effects produced by the dopamine receptor agonist at the supersensitive dopamine receptor compared to the intact dopamine receptor. In case of the supersensitive dopamine receptor, each dopamine recognition site may be coupled to more than one biological effector unit, leading not only to a lower threshold dose for activation of the biological process but also to an increase of the maximal biological response

to obtain a threshold response as well as to an increase in the number of spare receptors. This would lead to a narrowing of the fraction of receptors that can be coupled to the biological effector mechanism. It seems possible that such changes in the postsynaptic receptor mechanisms could lead to the development of all or none phenomena (*Fuxe*, 1979). Such phenomena have in fact been observed when Parkinsonian patients are chronically treated with large doses of l-DOPA (see *Rinne*, 1978). Thus, patients can switch from marked akinesia into hyperkinesia. The mechanism for such an effect could be the marked narrowing of the working range of the coupled DA receptors. The molecular basis for such a narrowing in the number of coupled receptors could be a reduction in synthesis of receptors and of coupling proteins induced by the excessive amounts of DA formed from l-DOPA.

References

Baldessarini, R. J.: The pathophysiological basis of tardive dyskinesia. Trends Neurosci. *2*, 133—135 (1979).

Birkmayer, W., Hornykiewicz, O.: Der L-Dioxyphenylalanin(L-DOPA-)-Effekt beim Parkinson-Syndrom des Menschen. Arch. Psychiat. Nervenkr. *203*, 560—574 (1962).

Birkmayer, W., Linauer, W., Mentasti, M., Riederer, P.: Zweijährige Erfahrungen mit einer Kombinationsbehandlung des Parkinson-Syndroms mit L-DOPA und dem Decarboxylasehemmer Benserazid (Ro 4-4602). Wien. med. Wschr. *124*, 340—344 (1974).

Burt, D. R., Creese, I., Snyder, S. H.: Properties of ³H-haloperidol and ³H-dopamine binding associated with dopamine receptors in calf brain membranes. Molec. Pharmacol. *12*, 631—638 (1976 a).

Burt, D. R., Creese, I., Snyder, S. H.: Properties of ³H-haloperidol and ³H-dopamine binding associated with dopamine receptors in calf brain membranes. Molec. Pharmacol. *12*, 800—812 (1976 b).

Calne, D. B., Plotkin, C., Williams, A. C., Nutt, J. G., Neophytides, A., Teychenne, P. F.: Long-term treatment of parkinsonism with bromocriptine. Lancet *1*, 735—738 (1978).

Calne, D. B., Teychenne, P. F., Claveria, L. E., Eastman, R., Greenacre, J. K., Petrie, A.: Bromocriptine in Parkinsonism. Br. Med. J. *4*, 442—444 (1974).

Cotzias, G. C., van Woert, M. H., Schiffer, L. M.: Aromatic amino acids and modification of Parkinsonism. New Engl. J. Med. *276*, 374—379 (1967).

Corrodi, H., Fuxe, K., Hökfelt, T., Lidbrink, P., Ungerstedt, U.: Effects of ergot drugs on central neurones: evidence for a stimulation of central dopamine neurons. J. Pharm. Pharmac. *25*, 409—412 (1973).

Creese, I., Burt, D. R., Snyder, S. H.: Dopamine receptor binding enhancement accompanies lesion-induced behavioural supersensitivity. Science *197*, 596—598 (1977).

Fuxe, K.: Tools in the treatment of Parkinson's disease: Studies on new types of dopamine receptor stimulating agents. In: Advances in Neurology (*Calne, D. B.,* ed.), pp. 273—279. New York: Raven Press. 1973.

Fuxe, K.: Dopamine receptor agonists in brain research and as therapeutic agents. Trends Neurosci. *2,* 1—4 (1979).

Fuxe, K., Corrodi, H., Hökfelt, T., Lidbrink, P., Ungerstedt, U.: Ergocornine and 2-Br-α-ergocryptine evidence for prolonged dopamine receptor stimulation. Med. Biol. *52,* 121—132 (1974).

Fuxe, K., Fredholm, B. B., Agnati, L. F., Ögren, S.-O., Everitt, B. J., Jonsson, G., Gustafsson, J.-Å.: Interaction of ergot drugs with central monoamine systems. Pharmacology *16,* Suppl. 1, 99—134 (1978 a).

Fuxe, K., Fredholm, B. B., Ögren, S.-O., Agnati, L. F., Hökfelt, T., Gustafsson, J.-Å.: Ergot drugs and central monoaminergic mechanisms: a histochemical, biochemical and behavioural analysis. Federation Proc. *37,* 2181—2191 (1978 b).

Fuxe, K., Ögren, S.-O., Agnati, L. F., Andersson, K., Hall, H., Köhler, C., Fredholm, B. B.: Central monoamine synapses as sites of action for ergot drugs. In: Ergot Alkaloids. New York: Raven Press. In press, 1979 a.

Fuxe, K., Schwarcz, R., Agnati, L. F., Fredholm, B. B., Ögren, S.-O., Köhler, C., Gustafsson, J.-Å.: Actions of ergot derivatives at dopamine synapses. In: Dopaminergic Ergot Derivatives and Motor Function (*Fuxe, K., Calne, D. B.,* eds.), pp. 151—157. Oxford: Pergamon Press. 1979 b.

Goldstein, M., Lew, J. Y., Nakamura, S., Battista, A. F., Lieberman, A., Fuxe, K.: Dopaminephilic properties of ergot alkaloids. Federation Proc. *37,* No. 8, 2202—2205 (1978).

Hökfelt, T., Fuxe, K.: On the morphology and the neuroendocrine role of the hypothalamic catecholamine neurons. In: Brain-Endocrine Interaction, Median Eminence: Structure and Function (*Knigge, K. M., Scott, D. E., Weindl, A.,* eds.), pp. 181—223. Basel: Karger. 1972.

Hollenberg, M. D.: Receptor models and the action of neurotransmitters and hormones. In: Neurotransmitter Receptor Binding (*Yamamura, H. I., Enna, S. J., Kuhar, M. J.,* eds.), pp. 13—39. New York: Raven Press. 1978.

Hornykiewicz, O.: The mechanisms of action of L-dopa in Parkinson's disease. Life Sci. *15,* 1249—1259 (1974).

Johnson, A. M., Loew, D. M., Bigouret, J. M.: Stimulant properties of bromocriptine on central dopamine receptors in comparison to apomorphine, (+)-amphetamine and L-dopa. Brit. J. Pharmacol. *56,* 59—68 (1976).

Lieberman, A. N., Kupersmith, M., Gopinathan, G., Estey, E., Goldstein, M.: Modification of the "on-off" effect with bromocriptine and lergotrile. In: Dopaminergic Ergot Derivatives and Motor Function (*Fuxe, K., Calne, D. B.,* eds.), pp. 285—295. Oxford: Pergamon Press. 1979.

Lieberman, A., Zolfaghari, M., Boal, D., Hassouri, H., Vogen, B., Battista, A., Fuxe, K., Goldstein, M.: The antiparkinsonian efficacy of bromocriptine. Neurology 26, 405—409 (1976).

Ludin, H. P., Bass-Verrey, F.: Study of deterioration in long-term treatment of parkinsonism with L-dopa plus decarboxylase inhibitor. J. Neural Transm. 38, 249—258 (1976).

Markstein, R., Herrling, P. L., Bürki, H. R., Asper, H., Ruch, W.: The effect of bromocriptine on the adenylate cyclase and the catecholamine metabolism of the rat brain. J. Neurochem. 31, 1163—1172 (1978).

Marsden, C. D., Parkes, J. D.: "On-off" effects in patients with Parkinson's disease on chronic levodopa therapy. Lancet 1, 292—296 (1976).

Marsden, C. D., Parkes, J. D.: Success and problems of long-term levodopa therapy in Parkinson's disease. Lancet 1, 345—349 (1977).

Miyamoto, T., Battista, A., Goldstein, M., Fuxe, K.: Long-lasting anti-tremor activity induced by 2-Br-α-ergocryptine in monkeys. J. Pharm. Pharmac. 26, 452—454 (1974).

Ögren, S.-O., Köhler, C., Fuxe, K., Ängeby, K.: Behavioural effects of ergot drugs. In: Dopaminergic Ergot Derivatives and Motor Function (*Fuxe, K., Calne, D. B.,* eds.), pp. 187—205. Oxford: Pergamon Press. 1979.

Parkes, J. D., de Bono, A. G., Marsden, C. D.: Bromocriptine in Parkinsonism, long-term treatment, dose response and comparison with levodopa. J. Neurol. Neurosurg. Psychiat. 39, 1101—1108 (1976).

Rinne, U. K.: Recent advances in research on Parkinsonism. Acta Neurol. Scand. 57, Suppl. 67, 77—113 (1978).

Schwarcz, R., Fuxe, K., Agnati, L. F., Gustafsson, J.-Å.: Effects of bromocriptine on ^{3}H-spiroperidol binding sites in rat striatum. Evidence for actions on dopamine receptors not linked to adenylate cyclase. Life Sci. 23, 465—470 (1978).

Schwarcz, R., Fuxe, K., Agnati, L. F., Hökfelt, T., Coyle, J. T.: Rotational behaviour in rats with unilateral striatal kainic acid lesions: A behavioural model for studies on intact dopamine receptors. Brain Res. 170, 485—495 (1979).

Trabucchi, M., Spano, P. F., Tonon, G. C., Frattola, L.: Effects of bromocriptine on central dopaminergic receptors. Life Sci. 19, 225—232 (1976).

Ungerstedt, U., Arbuthnott, G. W.: Quantitative recording of rotational behaviour in rats after 6-OH dopamine lesions of the nigrostriatal dopamine system. Brain Res. 24, 485—493 (1970).

Authors' address: Prof. Dr. *K. Fuxe,* Department of Histology, Karolinska Institutet, S-104 01 Stockholm 60, Sweden.

Journal of Neural Transmission, Suppl. 16, 83—93 (1980)

Contributions of α-Adrenoreceptor Blockade to Extrapyramidal Effects of Neuroleptic Drugs

N.-E. Andén and Maria Grabowska-Andén

Department of Medical Pharmacology, University of Uppsala, Uppsala, Sweden

Summary

Prazosin, phenoxybenzamine and clozapine, but not sulpiride, abolished the increase in flexor reflex activity induced by clonidine and they accelerated the noradrenaline utilization in the brain of rats. These findings indicate that the first three drugs block central α-adrenoreceptors. The α-methyltyrosine-induced disappearance of dopamine in the corpus striatum and the limbic system was decelerated by prazosin and phenoxybenzamine, was accelerated by sulpiride and was not significantly changed by clozapine. Prazosin and phenoxybenzamine almost completely reversed the sulpiride-induced increase in dopamine utilization. The reduction of the dopamine release following blockade of postsynaptic α-adrenoreceptors might prevent tardive dyskinesia. Blockade of postsynaptic α-adrenoreceptors might also increase the ultimate result of dopamine receptor stimulation in the corpus striatum but decrease that in the limbic system. Therefore, blockade of α-adrenoreceptors as well as of muscarinic receptors might explain why clozapine causes less extrapyramidal disturbances than other antipsychotic drugs.

Introduction

Clozapine differs from other neuroleptic drugs in the sense that it produces less parkinsonism or acute dystonia and less tardive dyskinesia both in animals and man (*Stille* and *Hippius*, 1971; *Hippius*, 1976; *Gunne* and *Bárány*, 1979). The absence of parkinsonism might be due to the clozapine-induced blockade of muscarinic receptors (*Andén* and *Stock*, 1973; *Snyder et al.*, 1974; *Miller* and *Hiley*, 1974). The anticholinergic effect of clozapine cannot, however, explain why tardive dyskinesia is not evoked since this condition often is worsened by muscarinic receptor blocking agents (*Crane*, 1972). Furthermore, a combination of haloperidol and a muscarinic receptor blocking agent is not able to reproduce all effects of clozapine in animal experiments, giving additional evidence for the view that the anticholinergic properties cannot be totally responsible for the lack of extrapyramidal manifestations following treatment with clozapine (*Bunney* and *Aghajanian*, 1976; *Sayers et al.*, 1976).

Clozapine also differs from other neuroleptic drugs by its relatively strong blockade of α-adrenoreceptors (*Stille et al.*, 1971). Therefore, we have given the two centrally active α-adrenoreceptor blocking agents prazosin and phenoxybenzamine (*Andén et al.*, 1978) in combination with a pure dopamine (DA) receptor blocking agent, sulpiride, and the effects of these combinations have been compared with those of clozapine. Clozapine and sulpiride have been administered to rats intraperitoneally at the doses 10 and 30 mg/kg, respectively. These doses cause a supramaximal blockade of post-synaptic DA receptors in the corpus striatum without any interference with the presynaptic DA receptors (*Andén* and *Grabowska-Andén*, 1979; *Andén* and *Grabowska-Andén*, 1980).

Materials and Methods

Male Sprague-Dawley rats weighing 155—270 g were used. Care was taken to keep the rectal temperature at 37 °C.

Flexor reflex activity. Clonidine increases flexor reflex activity by a stimulation of postsynaptic α-adrenoreceptors in the spinal cord (*Andén et al.*, 1970). The effects of prazosin, phenoxybenzamine, clozapine and sulpiride on the increase in hindlimb flexor reflex activity induced by clonidine (0.4 mg/kg i.p., 30 min after the other drugs) were studied in rats depleted of catecholamines and spinalized. The depletion was produced by reserpine (10 mg/kg i.p., 6 hours before the injection of clonidine). The spinal cord was transected at T2—T4 during diethylether anaesthesia about 1 hour after the injection of reserpine. The force and magnitude of the withdrawals of the hindlegs following a standardized pinching of the hindfeet were evaluated 60 min after the injection of clonidine. The changes were semiquantitatively estimated as 0 (no increase), 0.5 (small increase), 1 (clear-cut increase), 2 (marked increase), or 3 (maximal increase).

Utilization of Dopamine and Noradrenaline. The utilizations of DA and noradrenaline (NA) were investigated by means of the tyrosine hydro-xylase inhibitor DL-α-methyltyrosine methylester HCl (α-MT; 250 mg/kg i.p., 4 hours before sacrifice) (*Spector et al.*, 1965; *Corrodi* and *Hanson*, 1966; *Andén et al.*, 1966 a). The rats were killed by thoracotomy and ex-sanguination during light dichloromethane anaesthesia. The brain was quickly removed and placed on an ice-cooled Petri dish. Under an operation microscope, the brain was divided into the corpus striatum, the limbic system and the rest of the brain by sections at the lateral borders of the corpus striatum, through the internal capsules, at the frontal part of the optic chiasm, and through the rhinal fissures (*Andén et al.*, 1966 b). The DA (*Atack*, 1973) and the NA (*Bertler et al.*, 1958; *Häggendal*, 1963) were determined spectrofluorimetrically following homogenization in 0.4 N perchloric acid, cation exchange chromatography (*Atack* and *Magnusson*, 1970) and oxidation. The NA values in the corpus striatum are not reported due to the fact that they are very low and uncertain.

Drugs. The following drugs were used: reserpine (CIBA-Geigy*, Mölndal), clozapine (Sandoz*, Basle), sulpiride (Delagrange*, Paris), phenoxybenzamine HCl (SKF*, Philadelphia, Penn.), prazosin HCl (Pfizer*, Sandwich, Kent), clonidine HCl (Boehringer Ingelheim*, Stockholm), DL-α-methyltyrosine methylester HCl (α-MT, H 44/68; Hässle*, Mölndal). Reserpine, clozapine, sulpiride, phenoxybenzamine and prazosin were dissolved in a few drops of glacial acetic acid and the volume was made up with 5.5 % glucose. The doses refer to the forms indicated above.

Results

Flexor Reflex Activity

Clonidine (0.4 mg/kg i.p.) submaximally increased hindlimb flexor reflex activity of rats spinalized and depleted of catecholamines (Table 1). Prazosin, phenoxybenzamine, clozapine and sulpiride did not change the small normal flexor reflex tested before the injection

Table 1. *Effects of clozapine (10 mg/kg i.p.), sulpiride (30 mg/kg i.p.), phenoxybenzamine (30 mg/kg i.p.) and prazosin (10 mg/kg i.p.) on the clonidine-induced increase in hindlimb flexor reflex activity of rats. Clonidine (0.4 mg/kg i.p.) was given 30 min after the other drugs and 60 min before the evaluation of the reflex activity. The rats were pretreated with reserpine (10 mg/kg i.p.) and spinalized about 6 and 5 hours before clonidine, respectively. The number of rats is given in parentheses.The statistical significances were calculated using two-tailed Mann-Whitney U-test*

Treatment	Increase in flexor reflex activity*	Difference from clonidine controls
Clonidine	3 (4), 2 (1)	—
Prazosin + Clonidine	0 (5)	P < 0.008
Phenoxybenzamine + Clonidine	0.5 (2), 0 (3)	P < 0.008
Clozapine + Clonidine	1 (2), 0.5 (3)	P < 0.008
Sulpiride + Clonidine	3 (4), 2 (1)	P > 0.1

* 3 = maximal increase, 2 = marked increase, 1 = clearcut increase, 0.5 = small increase, 0 = no increase.

Table 2. *Concentrations of dopamine and noradrenaline in the corpus striatum, the limbic system and the rest of the brain of rats following treatment with clozapine (10 mg/kg i.p., $4^{1}/_4$ hours before sacrifice), sulpiride (30 mg/kg i.p., $4^{1}/_4$ hours), α-methyltyrosine methylester (α-MT, 250 mg/kg i.p., 4 hours), prazosin (10 mg/kg i.p., $4^{1}/_2$ hours) and phenoxybenzamine (30 mg/kg i.p., $4^{1}/_2$ hours). The values (mean ± S.E.M.) are per cent of untreated controls with the number of determinations in parentheses. The absolute concentrations of the untreated controls are shown in parentheses. The statistical significances were calculated using two-tailed Student's t-test*

Treatment	Dopamine corpus striatum	Dopamine limbic system	Dopamine rest of the brain	Noradrenaline limbic system	Noradrenaline rest of the brain
A. No drug treatment	100 ± 5.1 (6) (4.81 µg/g)	100 ± 4.7 (6) (0.827 µg/g)	100 ± 5.5 (6) (0.042 µg/g)	100 ± 5.8 (6) (0.427 µg/g)	100 ± 11.6 (6) (0.348 µg/g)
B. Clozapine	95 ± 10.8 (5) (B–A: P > 0.05)	87 ± 2.1 (5) (B–A: P < 0.05)	98 ± 9.8 (5) (B–A: P > 0.05)	76 ± 6.7 (5) (B–A: P < 0.025)	83 ± 7.2 (5) (B–A: P > 0.05)
C. Sulpiride	85 ± 4.8 (5) (C–A: P > 0.05)	69 ± 3.8 (5) (C–A: P < 0.001)	101 ± 9.5 (5) (C–A: P > 0.05)	84 ± 2.9 (5) (C–A: P < 0.05)	85 ± 4.2 (5) (C–A: P > 0.05)
D. α-MT	26 ± 1.2 (10) (D–A: P < 0.001)	23 ± 1.1 (10) (D–A: P < 0.001)	24 ± 2.9 (10) (D–A: P < 0.001)	58 ± 3.0 (10) (D–A: P < 0.001)	42 ± 1.8 (10) (D–A: P < 0.001)
E. Prazosin + α-MT	36 ± 5.0 (6) (E–D: P < 0.025)	29 ± 1.8 (6) (E–D: P < 0.01)	25 ± 3.8 (6) (E–D: P > 0.05)	33 ± 1.7 (6) (E–D: P < 0.001)	22 ± 1.4 (6) (E–D: P < 0.001)

F. Phenoxybenzamine + α-MT	38 ± 3.1 (6) (F–D: P < 0.001)	35 ± 3.1 (6) (F–D: P < 0.001)	20 ± 1.7 (6) (F–D: P > 0.05)	36 ± 1.8 (6) (F–D: P < 0.001)	15 ± 1.9 (6) (F–D: P < 0.001)
G. Clozapine + α-MT	29 ± 3.0 (6) (G–D: P > 0.05)	20 ± 1.3 (6) (G–D: P > 0.05)	29 ± 3.3 (6) (G–D: P > 0.05)	41 ± 2.8 (6) (G–D: P < 0.005)	22 ± 2.2 (6) (G–D: P < 0.001)
H. Sulpiride + α-MT	17 ± 1.4 (6) (H–D: P < 0.001)	13 ± 2.1 (6) (H–D: P < 0.001)	20 ± 2.9 (6) (H–D: P > 0.05)	43 ± 3.2 (6) (H–D: P < 0.01)	37 ± 2.7 (6) (H–D: P > 0.05)
I. Prazosin + Clozapine + α-MT	34 ± 2.6 (6) (I–E: P > 0.05) (I–G: P > 0.05)	27 ± 1.9 (6) (I–E: P > 0.05) (I–G: P < 0.025)	27 ± 3.6 (6) (I–E: P > 0.05) (I–G: P < 0.05)	27 ± 3.3 (6) (I–E: P > 0.05) (I–G: P < 0.01)	17 ± 1.6 (6) (I–E: P < 0.05) (I–G: P > 0.05)
K. Phenoxybenzamine + Clozapine + α-MT	37 ± 1.8 (6) (K–F: P > 0.05) (K–G: P < 0.05)	27 ± 2.0 (6) (K–F: P > 0.05) (K–G: P < 0.025)	29 ± 5.2 (6) (K–F: P > 0.05) (K–G: P > 0.05)	28 ± 3.6 (6) (K–F: P > 0.05) (K–G: P < 0.025)	14 ± 1.8 (6) (K–F: P > 0.05) (K–G: P < 0.025)
L. Prazosin + Sulpiride + α-MT	31 ± 1.7 (6) (L–E: P > 0.05) (L–H: P < 0.001)	22 ± 2.3 (6) (L–E: P < 0.05) (L–H: P < 0.025)	28 ± 2.1 (6) (L–E: P > 0.05) (L–H: P < 0.05)	26 ± 2.8 (6) (L–E: P < 0.05) (L–H: P < 0.005)	19 ± 2.6 (6) (L–E: P > 0.05) (L–H: P < 0.001)
M. Phenoxybenzamine + Sulpiride + α-MT	27 ± 1.8 (5) (M–F: P < 0.025) (M–H: P < 0.005)	21 ± 0.7 (5) (M–F: P < 0.005) (M–H: P < 0.01)	23 ± 5.5 (5) (M–F: P > 0.05) (M–H: P > 0.05)	27 ± 3.1 (5) (M–F: P < 0.05) (M–H: P < 0.01)	14 ± 1.6 (5) (M–F: P > 0.05) (M–H: P < 0.001)

of clonidine. The clonidine-induced increase in flexor reflex activity was blocked by prazosin (10 mg/kg i.p.) and phenoxybenzamine (30 mg/kg i.p.). It was almost completely inhibited by clozapine (10 mg/kg i.p.) but not at all by sulpiride (30 mg/kg i.p.).

Utilization of Dopamine

The α-MT-induced disappearance of DA in the corpus striatum and in the limbic system was decelerated by prazosin (10 mg/kg i.p.) and phenoxybenzamine (30 mg/kg i.p.) (Table 2). It was not significantly changed by clozapine (10 mg/kg i.p.). The DA was, however, higher (P < 0.025, Student's t-test) in the corpus striatum than in the limbic system following the combined treatment with clozapine and α-MT. On the other hand, sulpiride accelerated the utilization of DA in the corpus striatum and in the limbic system. In the rest of the brain, the α-MT-induced disappearance of DA did not appear to be significantly influenced by prazosin, phenoxybenzamine, clozapine and sulpiride.

The sulpiride-induced acceleration of the DA utilization in the corpus striatum and in the limbic system was almost completely antagonized by prazosin and phenoxybenzamine. The utilization of DA following clozapine was not changed to any great extent by prazosin and phenoxybenzamine.

Utilization of Noradrenaline

The α-MT-induced disappearance of NA was markedly accelerated by prazosin, phenoxybenzamine and clozapine but not by sulpiride (Table 2).

Discussion

The almost complete inhibition of the clonidine-induced increase in flexor reflex activity by clozapine indicates that this compound blocks postsynaptic α-adrenoreceptors to almost the same degree as prazosin and phenoxybenzamine. Sulpiride seems to lack effect on α-adrenoreceptors. The clozapine-induced increase in the utilization of NA might also be due to blockade of α-adrenoreceptors as suggested previously (Bartholini et al., 1972; Bürki et al., 1974; McMillen and Shore, 1978). The localization of the α-adrenoreceptors involved in this action is not clear since the turnover of NA is increased both following postsynaptic as well as presynaptic α-adreno-receptor blockade by, e.g. prazosin and yohimbine, respectively (Andén et al., 1976; Andén et al., 1978).

It has been hypothesized that the DA neurons to the corpus striatum are stimulated by increased postsynaptic α-adrenoreceptor activity in the brain to judge from data obtained by means of yohimbine, phenoxybenzamine and clonidine (*Andén* and *Grabowska*, 1976). Therefore, the postsynaptic α-adrenoreceptor blocking agents prazosin and phenoxybenzamine should reduce the activity of the nigro-neostriatal DA neurons. The inhibition of the DA utilization in the corpus striatum by these drugs might be caused by such a mechanism. The deceleration of the α-MT-induced disappearance of DA in the limbic system by prazosin and phenoxybenzamine suggests that there is a similar coupling between α-adrenoreceptors and the DA neurons to this area. The absence of effect of prazosin and phenoxy-benzamine on the turnover of DA in the brain outside the corpus striatum and the limbic system might indicates that this mechanism operates only in these two regions.

The sulpiride-induced acceleration of the α-MT-induced disappearance of DA is in all probability due to blockade of DA receptors since this dose of sulpiride supramaximally blocks the rotation induced by apomorphine following unilateral inactivation of the corpus striatum (*Andén* and *Grabowska-Andén*, 1980). The inhibitions by prazosin and phenoxybenzamine of the effect of sulpiride on the turnover of DA indicate that also the enhanced activity of the DA neurons can be slowed down by blockade of post-synaptic α-receptors. It should be noted that the dose of sulpiride used blocks only postsynaptic DA receptors (*Andén* and *Grabowska-Andén*, 1980). In preliminary experiments, the acceleration of the DA utilization following preferential blockade of presynaptic DA receptors by metoclopramide was not antagonized by blockade of postsynaptic α-adrenoreceptors.

The postsynaptic DA receptors in the corpus striatum are supra-maximally blocked by 10 mg/kg clozapine and 30 mg/kg sulpiride without any detectable blockade of the presynaptic DA receptors (*Andén* and *Grabowska-Andén*, 1979; *Andén* and *Grabowska-Andén*, 1980). Therefore, the lack of acceleration of the DA utilization following clozapine, but not sulpiride, can be explained if a stimulation of the DA neurons expected from the blockade of the DA receptors is antagonized by another action of clozapine. Such a factor might be the blockade of postsynaptic α-adrenoreceptors. Another possibility is the anticholinergic property of clozapine (*Stille et al.*, 1971) since muscarinic receptor blocking agents can counteract the neuroleptic-induced increases in the DA turnover (*Andén* and *Bédard*, 1971). The somewhat higher concentration of DA in the limbic system than in the corpus striatum following combined treatment with clozapine and α-MT indicates that this drug differentially changes the DA turnover in the two regions in agreement with previous results (*Andén* and *Stock*, 1973; *Zivkovic et al.*, 1975; *Bartholini*, 1976).

An α-adrenoreceptor blockade might be of importance for some extrapyramidal effects of neuroleptic drugs in addition to a DA receptor blockade. A drug blocking both α-adrenoreceptors and DA receptors inhibits the DA neurotransmission both presynaptically and postsynaptically. Such a dual effect might be of importance to prevent the development of tardive dyskinesia since this condition should be dependent on release of DA.

A blockade of postsynaptic α-adrenoreceptors can probably also change the ultimate result of stimulation of postsynaptic DA receptors. Inhibition of NA transmission has been reported to facilitate the stereotyped behaviour induced by apomorphine and amphetamine (*Mogilnicka* and *Braestrup*, 1976; *Grabowska-Andén*, 1977). In contrast, inhibition of NA transmission has been reported to reduce motor activity, both normally and following apomorphine and amphetamine (*Randrup et al.*, 1963; *Svensson* and *Waldeck*, 1969; *Maj et al.*, 1972). The stereotypies and the motor activity are probably stimulated by DA mechanisms in the corpus striatum and the nucleus accumbens, respectively (*Jackson et al.*, 1975). A blockade of muscarinic receptors might also selectively potentiate the effect of postsynaptic DA receptor stimulation in the corpus striatum (*Andén*, 1972). Therefore, the blockades of α-adrenoreceptors and muscarinic receptors by clozapine should decrease the functional significance of DA receptor blockade within but not outside the corpus striatum. A preferential inhibition of the extrastriatal DA mechanisms might prevent the development of parkinsonism and tardive dyskinesia in antipsychotic therapy.

Acknowledgements

This work was supported by the Swedish Medical Research Council (B80-04X-502-16C). For generous gifts of drugs we thank the companies indicated by asterisks above. Skilful technical assistance was provided by Marie Lager.

References

Andén, N.-E.: Dopamine turnover in the corpus striatum and the limbic system after treatment with neuroleptic and anti-acetylcholine drugs. J. Pharm. Pharmacol. 24, 905—906 (1972).

Andén, N.-E., Bédard, P.: Influences of cholinergic mechanisms on the function and turnover of brain dopamine. J. Pharm. Pharmacol. 23, 460—462 (1971).

Andén, N.-E., Corrodi, H., Dahlström, A., Fuxe, K., Hökfelt, T.: Effects of tyrosine hydroxylase inhibition on the amine levels of central mono-amine neurons. Life Sci. *5*, 561—568 (1966 a).

Andén, N.-E., Corrodi, H., Fuxe, K., Hökfelt, B., Hökfelt, T., Rydin, C., Svensson, T.: Evidence for a central noradrenaline receptor stimulation by clonidine. Life Sci. *9*, 513—523 (1970).

Andén, N.-E., Fuxe, K., Hamberger, B., Hökfelt, T.: A quantitative study of the nigro-neostriatal dopamine neuron system in the rat. Acta physiol. scand. *67*, 306—312 (1966 b).

Andén, N.-E., Gomes, C., Persson, B., Trolin, G.: R 28935 and prazosin: effects on central and peripheral alpha-adrenoreceptor activity and on blood pressure. Naunyn-Schmiedeberg's Arch. Pharmacol. *302*, 299—306 (1978).

Andén, N.-E., Grabowska, M.: Pharmacological evidence for a stimulation of dopamine neurons by noradrenaline neurons in the brain. Eur. J. Pharmacol. *39*, 275—282 (1976).

Andén, N.-E., Grabowska-Andén, M.: Presynaptic and postsynaptic effects of dopamine receptor blocking agents. Adv. Neurol., Vol. 24, pp. 235 to 245. New York: Raven Press. 1979.

Andén, N.-E., Grabowska-Andén, M.: Drug effects on pre- and post-synaptic dopamine receptors. Adv. Psychopharmacol. New York: Raven Press. 1980 (in press).

Andén, N.-E., Grabowska, M., Strömbom, U.: Different alpha-adreno-receptors in the central nervous system mediating biochemical and functional effects of clonidine and receptor blocking agents. Naunyn-Schmiedeberg's Arch. Pharmacol. *292*, 43—52 (1976).

Andén, N.-E., Stock, G.: Effect of clozapine on the turnover of dopamine in the corpus striatum and in the limbic system. J. Pharm. Pharmacol. *25*, 346—348 (1973).

Atack, C. V.: The determination of dopamine by a modification of the trihydroxyindole fluorimetric assay. Br. J. Pharmacol. *48*, 699—714 (1973).

Atack, C. V., Magnusson, T.: Individual elution of noradrenaline (together with adrenaline), dopamine, 5-hydroxytryptamine and histamine from a single, strong cation exchange column, by means of mineral acid-organic solvent mixtures. J. Pharm. Pharmacol. *22*, 625—627 (1970).

Bartholini, G.: Differential effect of neuroleptic drugs on dopamine turnover in extrapyramidal and limbic system. J. Pharm. Pharmacol. *28*, 429—433 (1976).

Bartholini, G., Haefeli, W., Jalfre, M., Keller, H. H., Pletscher, A.: Effects of clozapine on cerebral catecholaminergic neurone systems. Br. J. Pharmacol. *46*, 736—740 (1972).

Bertler, Å., Carlsson, A., Rosengren, E.: A method for the fluorimetric determination af adrenaline and noradrenaline in tissues. Acta physiol. scand. *44*, 273—292 (1958).

Bunney, B. S., Aghajanian, G. K.: The effect of antipsychotic drugs on the firing of dopaminergic neurons: a reappraisal. In: Antipsychotic Drugs:

92   N.-E. Andén and Maria Grabowska-Andén:

Pharmacodynamics and Pharmacokinetics, pp. 305—318. Oxford: Pergamon Press. 1976.

Bürki, H. R., Ruch, W., Asper, H., Baggiolini, M., Stille, G.: Effect of single and repeated administration of clozapine on the metabolism of dopamine and noradrenaline in the brain of the rat. Eur. J. Pharmacol. *27*, 180 to 190 (1974).

Corrodi, H., Hanson, L. C. F.: Central effects of an inhibitor of tyrosine hydroxylation. Psychopharmacologia *10*, 116—125 (1966).

Crane, G. E.: Pseudoparkinsonism and tardive dyskinesia. Arch. Neurol. *27*, 426—430 (1972).

Grabowska-Andén, M.: Modification of the amphetamine-induced stereotypy in rats following inhibition of the noradrenaline release by FLA 136. J. Pharm. Pharmacol. *29*, 566—567 (1977).

Gunne, L.-M., Bárány, S.: A monitoring test for the liability of neuroleptic drugs to induce tardive dyskinesia. Psychopharmacology *63*, 195—198 (1979).

Häggendal, J.: An improved method for fluorimetric determination of small amounts of adrenaline and noradrenaline in plasma and tissues. Acta physiol. scand. *59*, 242—254 (1963).

Hippius, H.: On the relations between antipsychotic and extrapyramidal effects of psychoactive drugs. In: Antipsychotic Drugs: Pharmacodynamics and Pharmacokinetics, pp. 437—445. Oxford: Pergamon Press. 1976.

Jackson, D. M., Andén, N.-E., Dahlström, A.: A functional effect of dopamine in the nucleus accumbens and in some other dopamine-rich parts of the rat brain. Psychopharmacologia *45*, 139—149 (1975).

Maj, J., Grabowska, M., Gajda, L.: Effect of apomorphine on motility in rats. Eur. J. Pharmacol. *17*, 208—214 (1972).

McMillen, B. A., Shore, P. A.: Comparative effects of clozapine and α-adrenoceptor blocking drugs on regional noradrenaline metabolism in rat brain. Eur. J. Pharmacol. *52*, 225—230 (1978).

Miller, R. J., Hiley, C. R.: Anti-muscarinic properties of neuroleptics and drug-induced Parkinsonism. Nature *248*, 596—597 (1974).

Mogilnicka, E., Braestrup, C.: Noradrenergic influence on the stereotyped behaviour induced by amphetamine, phenethylamine and apomorphine. J. Pharm. Pharmacol. *28*, 253—255 (1975).

Randrup, A., Munkvad, I., Udsen, P.: Adrenergic mechanisms and amphetamine induced abnormal behaviour. Acta pharmacol. toxicol. *20*, 145—157 (1963).

Sayers, A. C., Bürki, H. R., Ruch, W., Asper, H.: Anticholinergic properties of antipsychotic drugs and their relation to extrapyramidal side-effects. Psychopharmacology *51*, 15—22 (1976).

Snyder, S. H., Banerjee, S. P., Yamamura, H. I., Greenberg, D.: Drugs, neurotransmitters and schizophrenia. Science *184*, 1243—1253 (1974).

Spector, S., Sjoerdsma, A., Udenfriend, S.: Blockade of endogenous norepinephrine synthesis by α-methyltyrosine, an inhibitor of tyrosine hydroxylase. J. Pharmacol. exp. Ther. *147*, 86—95 (1965).

Stille, G., Hippius, H.: Kritische Stellungnahme zum Begriff der Neuroleptika (anhand von pharmakologischen und klinischen Befunden mit Clozapin). Pharmacopsychiat. Neuro-Psychopharmacol. *4*, 182—191 (1971).

Stille, G., Lauener, H., Eichenberger, E.: The pharmacology of 8-chloro-11-(4-methyl-1-piperazinyl)-5H-dibenzo[b, e] [1, 4] diazepine (clozapine). Il. Farmaco, Ed. Pr. *26*, 605—625 (1971).

Svensson, T. H., Waldeck, B.: On the significance of central noradrenaline for motor activity: experiments with a new dopamine-β-hydroxylase inhibitor. Eur. J. Pharmacol. *7*, 278—282 (1969).

Zivkovic, B., Guidotti, A., Revuelta, A., Costa, E.: Effect of thioridazine, clozapine and other antipsychotics on the kinetic state of tyrosine hydroxylase and on the turnover rate of dopamine in striatum and nucleus accumbens. J. Pharmacol. exp. Ther. *194*, 37—46 (1975).

Authors' address: Dr. *N.-E. Andén*, Box 573, Biomedicum, S-751 23 Uppsala, Sweden.

Journal of Neural Transmission, Suppl. 16, 95—101 (1980)
© by Springer-Verlag 1980

The Decarboxylation of DOPA in the Parkinsonian Brain: *In vivo* Studies on an Animal Model

F. Hefti, E. Melamed, and R. J. Wurtman

Laboratory of Neuroendocrine Regulation, Department of Nutrition and Food Science, Massachusetts Institute of Technology, Cambridge, Massachusetts, U.S.A.

Summary

The site of decarboxylation of exogenously administered L-DOPA was studied in corpora striata of rats with near-total unilateral nigrostriatal lesions. After DOPA administration, the absolute increases in dopamine (DA) levels were lower in lesioned than in unlesioned striata, suggesting that, in the intact striatum, a major part of exogenous DOPA is decarboxylated in DA neurons. DOPA can also be decarboxylated outside DA neurons, however, as shown by our finding that relatively higher DOPA decarboxylase than tyrosine hydroxylase activity or DA concentration remains in striata after the nigrostriatal lesions. Also, the percentage increases in DA formation after DOPA administration were much higher in lesioned than in control striata. Rats with both raphé and nigrostriatal lesions failed to exhibit further reductions in striatal DOPA decarboxylase activity or diminished biochemical or behavioral (turning behavior) reactions to DOPA. Inhibition of the DOPA decarboxylase contained in brain capillary endothelial cells did not abolish DA formation in lesioned striata or circling behavior after DOPA administration. These findings all suggest an additional cell type in the striatum as the site of DOPA's decarboxylation in the absence of DA neurons.

Introduction

L-DOPA, the agent most widely used to treat Parkinson's disease, apparently acts by replenishing deficient striatal dopamine (DA) stores after being decarboxylated to DA by the enzyme L-aromatic amino decarboxylase (DOPA decarboxylase, DDC) (*Hornykiewicz,* 1974). Over long-term administration its therapeutic efficacy often declines gradually; it has been suggested that this decline is due to the continuous death of nigrostriatal neurons as Parkinson's disease progresses, reducing the enzymatic substrate for decarboxylation of exogenous DOPA (*Fahn* and *Calne,* 1978). However, other findings suggest that DOPA might be decarboxylated to DA outside DA neurons, in structures not primarily affected by Parkinson's disease, *i.e.,* in striatal serotoninergic (5-HT) neurons (*Ng et al.,* 1972) or in endothelial cells of brain capillaries (*Vogt,* 1970).

Given the important clinical implications of this question, we re-examined the site of exogenous DOPA decarboxylation in the parkinsonian brain, using rats with specific nigrostriatal lesions as models for human parkinsonism. Near-total lesions of the DA nigro-striatal tract were performed by injecting 6-hydroxydopamine into the substantia nigra and medial forebrain bundle. To assess the contribution of non-DA structures to exogenous DOPA decarboxyla-tion, additional lesions were performed or the rats were treated with a specific inhibitor to block DDC in blood vessels.

Decarboxylation of Exogenous DOPA in DA Neurons

In rats with unilateral nigrostriatal 6-hydroxydopamine lesions, L-DOPA caused large, dose-dependent increases in striatal DA con-centrations in both lesioned and unlesioned striata (Table 1), con-firming data obtained on cats with electrolytic lesions of the substantia nigra (*Langelier et al.,* 1973). The unlesioned side had larger absolute increases, suggesting that, in the intact striatum, a major fraction of exogenous DOPA is decarboxylated in DA neurons. Accordingly, DOPA levels were higher in the lesioned side, indicating that DA neurons used more DOPA in the intact striatum. Relative increases, however, were larger in the lesioned side; *e.g.,* 500 mg/kg L-DOPA increased DA concentrations 18-fold in the lesioned striatum, but only 3-fold in the contralateral side. If the DA neurons surviving 6-hydroxydopamine lesions were the sole DOPA decarboxylation site in lesioned striata, the relative increases in DA should have been the same on both sides. Our finding therefore confirms those of *Lytle et al.* (1972), that some additional striatal constituent decarboxylates DOPA after nigrostriatal lesions.

The concentrations of the DA metabolites dihydroxyphenylacetic acid (DOPAC) and homovanillic acid (HVA) were markedly enhanced to the same extent in lesioned and unlesioned striata after DOPA administration (Table 1). However, differences between the two sides appeared when DOPA was administered with carbidopa,

Table 1. *Formation of DA and its metabolites from exogenous DOPA in normal and 6-OHDA-lesioned striatum (ng/mg wet weight)*

Treatment	Side	DOPA	DA	DOPAC	HVA
Control (n = 6)	lesioned	n.d.	0.49±0.14[1]	0.14±0.05[1]	0.11±0.03[1]
	contralateral	n.d.	7.85±0.59	0.59±0.15	0.93±0.24
DOPA 100 mg/kg (n = 7)	lesioned	1.71±0.19[1]	2.37±0.40[1,2]	9.20±2.99[2]	4.04±0.56[2]
	contralateral	0.74±0.06	9.14±0.67	11.62±2.84[3]	5.33±1.30[3]
DOPA 500 mg/kg (n = 6)	lesioned	13.83±3.79[1]	7.76±1.48[1,2]	31.25±8.16[2]	6.53±1.14[2]
	contralateral	7.74±2.29	20.71±3.25[3]	34.50±5.66[3]	6.36±0.91[3]
DOPA 100 mg/kg + carbidopa (n = 8)	lesioned	20.04±1.95[1]	4.74±0.63[1,2,4]	4.73±1.21[1,2,4]	1.81±0.38[1,2,4]
	contralateral	8.12±0.94	19.13±1.86[3]	12.37±2.03[3]	3.74±1.10[3]

Data are expressed as means ± S.E.M. Rats (150 g) were injected unilaterally with 8 μg 6-OHDA into the substantia nigra and 4 μg in the medial forebrain bundle. Two weeks after lesioning, they were injected (i.p.) with carbidopa (100 mg per kg) and 60 min later with L-DOPA and were killed 45 min later. Striata were dissected and assayed for DOPA, DA, and DA metabolites (using high-performance liquid chromatography with electrochemical detection; *Felice et al.*, 1979; *Hefti*, 1979) and TH activity (*Waymire et al.*, 1971). TH activities and DA levels in the lesioned striatum of unlesioned rats were reduced to 5—10 % of those in the contralateral striatum. TH activities were used to assess the severity of lesions in DOPA-treated rats; in all groups, they were reduced to the same extent as in untreated rats.

[1] P < 0.05 differs from contralateral side.
[2] P < 0.01 differs from lesioned side of untreated rats.
[3] P < 0.01 differs from unlesioned side of untreated rats.
[4] P < 0.05 differs from lesioned side of rats given 500 mg/kg DOPA.

a peripheral DDC inhibitor: DOPAC and HVA reached significantly lower levels in the lesioned than in the contralateral side. Therefore, minor fractions of these metabolites are formed after release from DA neurons. Pretreatment with carbidopa decreased the DOPA-induced elevation of DOPAC and HVA concentrations in lesioned striata, suggesting that important fractions of these metabolites are derived from DOPA decarboxylation in blood vessels.

Our data show that most striatal DDC activity is localized in DA neurons. Lesions that reduce striatal DA levels and tyrosine hydroxylase (TH) activity to 5 % of control values reduced DDC activity to about 20 % (Table 2). The smaller relative reduction in DDC activity also indicates that some striatal structure other than nigrostriatal terminals contains this enzyme and might participate in DOPA decarboxylation.

DA formed from exogenous DOPA in DA neurons is likely to be released at the same sites as endogenous DA and can reach post-synaptic DA receptors. However, the same would not necessarily be true for DA formed in other striatal structures: thus it became important to test the functional effectiveness of DA formed outside DA neurons. Rats with unilateral nigrostriatal lesions respond to administration of DA agonists or L-DOPA with a characteristic rotational behavior, which is mediated by supersensitive DA receptors

Table 2. *Effect of various lesions on striatal TH and DDC activities*[1]

	TH	DDC
6-OHDA unilaterally (n = 16)	5.3 ± 1.7	19.7 ± 1.1[2]
6-OHDA unilaterally + raphé lesions (n = 6)	5.1 ± 0.9	21.0 ± 4.2[2]
6-OHDA unilaterally + kainic acid unilaterally (n = 6)	9.3 ± 4.4	11.2 ± 2.7

[1] Enzyme activities in the lesioned striatum are expressed as percentage of those in the contralateral side. Results are given as means $\pm$ S.E.M.

[2] Significantly smaller decrease than that in TH activity, $P < 0.001$.

Unilateral nigrostriatal lesions were produced by injecting rats with 8 μg 6-OHDA into the substantia nigra and 4 μg into the medial forebrain bundle. Raphé nuclei were lesioned electrolytically; these lesions reduced striatal serotonin content in both sides to 10 % of that in control rats (*Melamed et al.*, 1979). Kainic acid (2.5 μg) was injected into the same side as the 6-OHDA; these injections reduced striatal L-glutamate decarboxylase activity and substance P concentrations to 30 % of those in the contra-lateral side. Rats were killed two weeks after lesioning. Both enzyme activities were measured in portions of the same striatal homogenate (*McGeer et al.*, 1973; *Waymire et al.*, 1971).

in the lesioned striatum (*Ungerstedt*, 1969). Circling behavior after L-DOPA therefore reflects the functional effectiveness of DA formed in lesioned striata. In our study, all rats with lesions reducing striatal TH activity or DA levels to less than 10 % of control values showed vigorous turning behavior when injected with DOPA. No decrease in this response occurred in rats with TH activity and DA levels reduced below the limit of sensitivity of the methods used (below 1 % of control values), suggesting that DA formed from DOPA outside DA neurons is functionally effective.

Role of DOPA Decarboxylase in Brain Capillaries

The endothelial cells of brain capillaries contain DDC and can decarboxylate DOPA (*Bertler et al.*, 1966). Accordingly, part of the increased DA concentration that we observed after DOPA administration may have reflected formation in capillaries. We compared a group of lesioned rats injected with 100 mg/kg L-DOPA plus an inhibitor of peripheral DDC (carbidopa) with another group given 500 mg/kg L-DOPA, *i.e.*, treatments that similarly elevate brain DOPA levels (Table 1), and found reduced DA formation after inhibition of peripheral DDC (Table 1). However, pretreatment with carbidopa did not prevent large increases in DA concentration in the lesioned striatum; the large discrepancy between the relative increases in the unlesioned and lesioned sides remained. Furthermore, carbidopa failed to prevent or reduce the DOPA-induced circling behavior, confirming the results of *Duvoisin* and *Mytilineou* (1978), thus suggesting that DA formed in blood vessels does not contribute significantly to striatal DA's functional effectiveness.

Role of Serotoninergic Neurons

Large doses of L-DOPA decrease brain 5-HT levels; this action probably reflects 5-HT's displacement by DA formed from exogenously administered DOPA in 5-HT neurons, a mechanism that occurs *in vitro* (*Ng et al.*, 1972). *Ng et al.* (1972) therefore proposed that DA itself could be released from striatal 5-HT terminals after DOPA administration and reach the postsynaptic DA receptors. We tested this hypothesis by inducing lesions in the raphé nuclei of rats with nigrostriatal lesions. Additional raphé lesions did not reduce formation of DA and its metabolites or suppress circling behavior after DOPA administration (*Melamed et al.*, 1979). Furthermore, raphé lesions did not reduce striatal DDC activity or abolish the difference between the relative decreases in TH and DDC activities observed after nigrostriatal lesions (Table 2). These findings do not favor the view that 5-HT neurons contribute significantly to DA formation from exogenous DOPA in the striatum.

Decarboxylation in Other Striatal Cells

DOPA decarboxylation outside of DA neurons could also theoretically occur in glial or any other neuronal cells in the striatum. We injected kainic acid (a neurotoxin primarily destroying neuronal cell bodies and inducing massive glial proliferation; *Schwarcz* and *Coyle*, 1977) into striata of rats with ipsilateral nigrostriatal lesions. Such combined lesions tended to reduce striatal DDC activity even further than did 6-hydroxydopamine lesions alone and abolished the difference between the relative reductions in TH and DDC activities (Table 2). This finding favors a neuronal system as additional source of striatal DDC activity and suggests that striatal glial cells do not contain a significant amount of this enzyme, since no increases in its activity were observed despite glial proliferation.

In conclusion, our study suggests that, in the intact striatum, a major part of exogenously administered DOPA is decarboxylated in DA neurons. An additional striatal structure (most likely not 5-HT neurons, blood vessels, or glial cells) contains DDC capable of converting exogenously administered DOPA to functionally effective DA in the absence of DA neurons. By inference, the frequent decline of DOPA's efficacy in treating Parkinson's disease apparently does not result from loss of the enzymatic substrate for DOPA decarboxylation caused by continuous degeneration of DA neurons.

References

Bertler, A., Falck, B., Owman, C., Rosengren, E.: The localization of mono-aminergic blood-brain barrier mechanisms. Pharmacol. Rev. *18*, 369—385 (1966).

Duvoisin, R. C., Mytilineou, C.: Where is L-DOPA decarboxylated after 6-hydroxydopamine nigrotomy? Brain Res. *152*, 369—373 (1978).

Fahn, S., Calne, M. L.: Considerations in the management of parkinsonism. Neurology *28*, 5—7 (1978).

Felice, L. J., Felice, J. D., Kissinger, P. T.: Determination of catecholamines in rat brain parts by reverse-phase ion-pair liquid chromatography. J. Neurochem. *31*, 1461—1466 (1978).

Hefti, F.: A simple, sensitive method for measuring 3, 4-dihydroxyphenyl-acetic acid and homovanillic acid in rat brain tissue using high-performance liquid chromatography with electrochemical detection. Life Sci. *25,* 775—782 (1979).

Hornykiewicz, O.: The mechanism of action of L-DOPA in Parkinson's disease. Life Sci. *15,* 1249—1259 (1974).

Langelier, P., Roberge, A. G., Boucher, R., Poirier, L. J.: Effects of chronically administered L-DOPA in normal and lesioned cats. J. Pharmacol. Exp. Ther. *187,* 15—26 (1973).

Lytle, L. D., Hurko, O., Romero, J. A., Cottman, K., Leehey, D., Wurtman, R. J.: The effects of 6-hydroxydopamine pretreatment on the accumulation of DOPA and dopamine in brain and peripheral organs following L-DOPA administration. J. Neural Transm. *33,* 63—72 (1972).

McGeer, E. G., Fibiger, H. C., McGeer, P. L., Brooke, S.: Temporal changes in amine synthesizing enzymes of rat extrapyramidal structures after hemitranssections or 6-OHDA administration. Brain Res. *52,* 289—300 (1973).

Melamed, E., Hefti, F., Wurtman, R. J.: Decarboxylation of L-DOPA in Parkinson's disease. Is there a role for serotoninergic neurons? Submitted for publication.

Ng, L. K. Y., Chase, T. N., Colburn, R. W., Kopin, I. J.: L-DOPA in Parkinsonism; a possible mechanism of action. Neurology 22, 688—695 (1972).

Schwarcz, R., Coyle, J. T.: Striatal lesions with kainic acid; neurochemical characteristics. Brain Res. *127,* 235—250 (1977).

Ungerstedt, U.: Postsynaptic supersensitivity after 6-hydroxydopamine induced degeneration of nigrostriatal dopamine system. Acta Physiol. Scand., suppl. *367,* 69—93 (1971).

Vogt, M.: Drug-induced changes in brain dopamine and their relation to parkinsonism. Sci. Basis Med. Annu. Rev., chapter XVI, pp. 276—291 (1970).

Waymire, J. C., Bujn, R., Weiner, N.: Assay of tyrosine hydroxylase by coupled decarboxylation of dopa formed from l-^{14}C-tyrosine. Anal. Biochem. *43,* 588—600 (1971).

Authors' address: Prof. Dr. *R. J. Wurtman,* Laboratory of Neuroendocrine Regulation, 56-245, Massachusetts Institute of Technology, Cambridge, MA 02139, U.S.A.

Journal of Neural Transmission, Suppl. 16, 103—109 (1980)
© by Springer-Verlag 1980

Metabolic Alterations in an Animal Model of Huntington's Disease Using the ^{14}C-Deoxyglucose Method

H. Kimura, Edith G. McGeer, and P. L. McGeer

Kinsmen Laboratory of Neurological Research, Department of Psychiatry,
University of British Columbia, Vancouver, B.C., Canada

With 1 Figure

Summary

Various brain regions showing altered glucose uptake in an animal model of Huntington's disease (HD) were identified by the ^{14}C-2-deoxy-glucose (DG) autoradiographic technique. Rats with kainic acid (KA) lesions of the neostriatum were used as an animal model of HD. KA-injected animals showed reduced utilization of DG in the injected neostriatum as well as in the ipsilateral rostral sulcal cortex, dentate fascia of hippocampus, ventromedial nucleus of the thalamus and cortico-bulbar tract. By contrast, enhanced uptake was found in the ipsilateral globus pallidus, entopeduncular nucleus, the area lateral to the lateral hypothalamus, the lateral habenular nucleus and pars reticulata of the substantia nigra. The results provide interesting *in vivo* metabolic and functional information on brain circuits involved in motor performance.

The primary pathology important to the movement disorder in Parkinsonism, initially demonstrated by the work of Birkmayer and his colleagues, is a deficiency in the nigrostriatal dopaminergic tract, while postsynaptic structures in the neostriatum are spared. By contrast, the nigrostriatal dopaminergic system is relatively intact in Huntington's disease (HD), but there is a substantial loss of neurons in the caudate and putamen. The two disorders exhibit opposite features, those of dyskinesia in the former and chorea in the latter.

Selective destruction of the nigrostriatal system in rats can be produced by injections of 6-hydroxydopamine (6-OHDA) into the medial forebrain bundle while intrastriatal injections of kainic acid

(KA) produce pathological, biochemical and psychopharmacological changes very similar to those found in HD (*Coyle et al.*, 1978; *Fibiger*, 1978). Such selective neuronal losses presumably produce changes in the activity of other, interconnected nuclei and identification of such nuclei should cast new light on the mechanisms of movement control and, possibly, on the etiology of some of the other symptomatology seen in these basal ganglia disorders. The autoradiographic deoxyglucose technique developed by *Sokoloff* and his colleagues (1977) permits measurement of the relative glucose metabolism in various brain areas. *Schwartz et al.* (1976) applied this method to 6-OHDA-lesioned rats. This paper describes preliminary results in the application of this technique to animals with unilateral KA-induced lesions.

Materials and Methods

Male Wistar rats weighing approximately 300 grams were injected intrastriatally with 4 nmol of KA in 0.5 μl of phosphate buffered saline (*McGeer* and *McGeer*, 1978). These injections were done unilaterally under Nembutal anesthesia in a stereotaxic apparatus using coordinates from the *König* and *Klippel* (1963) atlas with suitable adjustments for animal weight. KA under the condition used here causes about 45—50 % destruction of neostriatal cholinergic and GABA-ergic neurons without significant effects on the dopaminergic efferents (*McGeer* and *McGeer*, 1978). A number of other intrinsic neuronal types in the striatum also seem to be destroyed by the KA injections (*Coyle et al.*, 1978). Nine days after the intracerebral injections, the injected and control rats were catheterized into the femoral vein under Nembutal anesthesia. In our previous experiments (*Kimura* and *Wada*, 1979), we found that the effect of Nembutal on the ^{14}C-deoxyglucose (DG) uptake by brain endures for at least six hours. Furthermore, the noxious stimulation inherent in the operational procedure also seems to affect the DG consumption. Therefore, we waited 24 hours before injecting 25 μCi of DG (specific activity 316 mCi/mmol) in 125 μl of 0.9 % saline into the cannula. Animals were sacrificed 45 min later by cervical fracture. The brains were sectioned with a cryostat and autoradiograms were prepared according to the method of *Sokoloff et al.* (1977). X-ray film (Kodak X-O mat R) was exposed against the sections for 7 days. After developing these films, the same sections were stained with cresyl violet for histological observation in order to confirm precise regions of interest as well as injection sites.

Results and Discussion

Autoradiograms of some coronal sections from KA-injected rats are shown in Fig. 1. The uninjected side of these rats showed no detectable differences compared to sections from control animals so that no contralateral effects of KA were seen with the present technique. As can be seen from Fig. 1, KA-injected animals showed reduced utilization of DG in the injected neostriatum as well as in the ipsilateral rostral sulcal cortex, dentate fascia of the hippocampus, ventromedial nucleus of the thalamus and cortico-bulbar tract. By contrast there was markedly enhanced uptake in the ipsilateral globus pallidus, entopeduncular nucleus, the area lateral to the lateral hypothalamus (probably corresponding to the substantia innominata in primates), the lateral habenular nucleus and the pars reticulata of the substantia nigra.

The results are striking in that some areas show sharply reduced metabolism, while others show considerably enhanced metabolism. They suggest which pathways may have dominant excitatory or inhibitory mechanisms in the dynamic loops associated with movement.

The reduced uptake in the injected neostriatum is not surprising in view of the local neuronal loss seen in histological studies (*Coyle et al.,* 1978) although no change in oxygen uptake was found in *in vitro* incubation of slices from KA-injected striata (*Jakubovic et al.,* 1979). This phenomenon may reflect the differing metabolism of neuronal and glial cells.

The greatly enhanced uptake in the pars reticulata of the substantia nigra might be connected with the loss of much of the descending inhibitory GABA-ergic input from the striatum. It has been reported that GABA is particularly concentrated in the pars reticulata (*Kanazawa* and *Toyokura,* 1975) and mainly originates from the striatum, via the strio-nigral pathway. Destruction of this pathway has been shown following intrastriatal KA injections (*Coyle et al.,* 1978). Similarly, enhanced uptake in the globus pallidus and entopeduncular nucleus could also be due to the loss of inhibitory striatal GABA inputs.

The decreased uptake in the ventromedial nucleus of the thalamus may reflect increased activity of the reportedly inhibitory input (*Anderson* and *Yoshida,* 1977) from the pars reticulata of the substantia nigra and/or a decrease in some unidentified excitatory input.

The results suggest that in the extrapyramidal loops that normally coordinate motor function, the descending strio-nigral and strio-pallidal pathways play predominantly inhibitory roles.

Several limbic structures were also affected. The decreased activity in the sulcal cortex, which includes the perirhinal and lateral entorhinal cortex, could be expected to produce decreased activity in the dentate gyrus of the hippocampus, since the perforant pathway

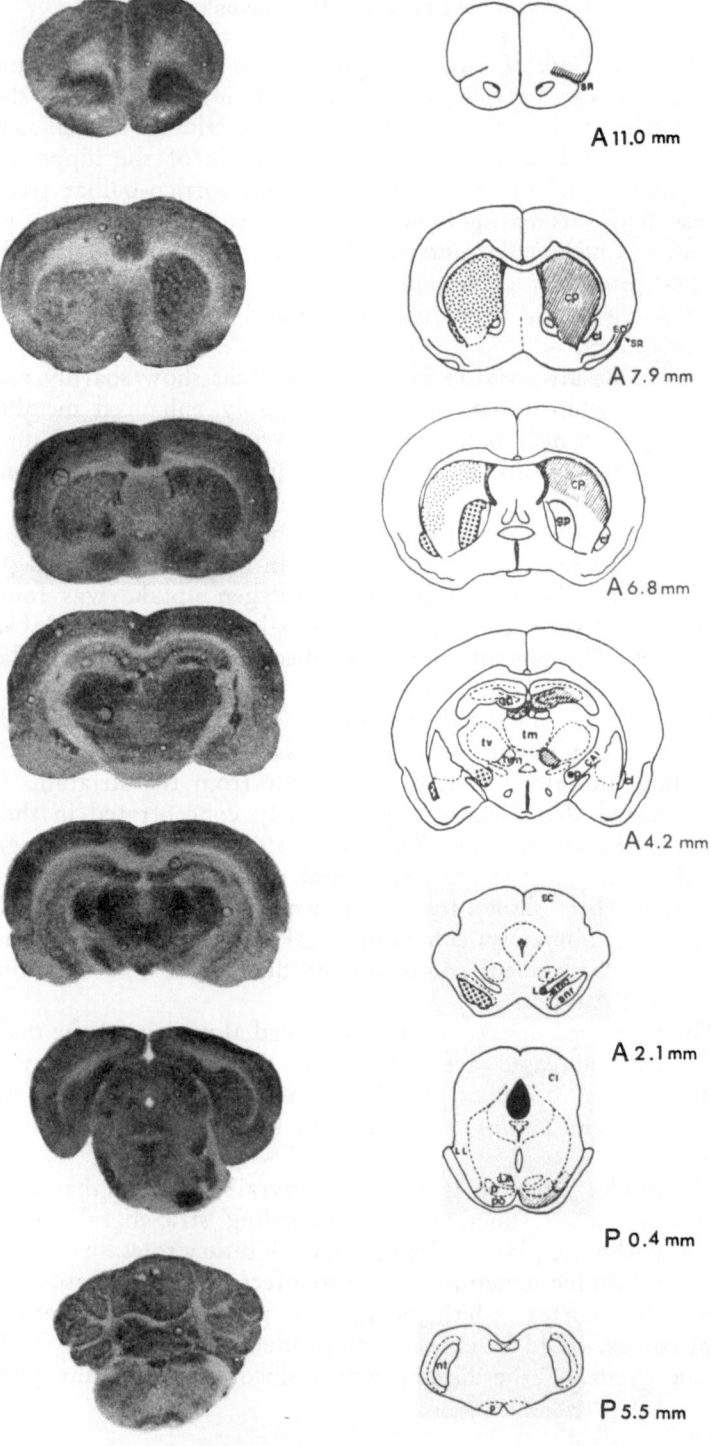

A 11.0 mm

A 7.9 mm

A 6.8 mm

A 4.2 mm

A 2.1 mm

P 0.4 mm

P 5.5 mm

connecting both areas is believed to use glutamate as the excitatory input to the hippocampus (*Nadler et al.*, 1976). The reason for the decrease in the sulcal cortex is not clear. It may be connected with a change in the dopaminergic innervation reported by *Burger et al.* (1976) to the rostral sulcal cortex (which is regarded as homologous with the primate prefrontal cortex) or result from a change in the thalamic projections to this area.

The increased activity in the habenular nucleus would suggest either that the dominant input from the entopeduncular nucleus is excitatory since the level of activity was also increased in that structure or that some other excitatory input was stimulated. Alternatively, an inhibitory pathway could have been knocked out by the KA injections, but this is unlikely to be the reported entopeduncular-(lateral)habenula pathway employing GABA (*Gottesfeld* and *Jakobowitz*, 1978) since increased rather than decreased uptake was also seen in the entopeduncular nucleus.

Reduced uptake of DG was also seen in the cortico-bulbar tract. This reduced activity could mean that fewer impulses were originating from the cortex, or that some axons of passage through the striatum were damaged by the injection. Changes in the cortico-spinal tract could not be detected although the animals showed circling behavior contralateral to the lesion.

Schwartz et al. (1976), using a similar technique following unilateral injections of 6-OHDA or electrolytic lesions to the medial forebrain bundle, reported decreased DG uptake in the cortex, striatum and thalamus. They did not apparently find any areas showing uptake increased over control.

The present results with DG following KA lesions provide interesting correlative *in vivo* metabolic and functional information

---

Fig. 1. Representative radioautograms and schematic diagrams after the *König* and *Klippel*'s atlas (1963). The left hemisphere is the KA-lesioned side. Open circles indicate the extent of the lesion in the neostriatum; closed circles indicate the increased uptake on the ipsilateral side of the lesion; shading on the contralateral side indicates these areas which appeared darker on that side than on the ipsilateral side. Since the uptake on the contralateral side appeared identical to that in controls, such shading identifies areas with decreased DG uptake on the side ipsilateral to the lesion. *a* nucleus accumbens; *CAI* capsula interna; *CI* colliculus inferior; *cl* claustrum; *cp* nucleus caudatus, putamen; *ep* nucleus entopeduncularis; *gp* globus pallidus; *GD* gyrus dentatus; *LL* lemniscus lateralis; *LM* lemniscus medialis; *nt* nuclei trigemini; *p* tractus corticospinalis; *po* nuclei pontis; *p* nucleus ruber; *SC* colliculus superior; *snc* substantia nigra zona compacta; *snr* substantia nigra zona reticularis; *SR* sulcus rhinalis; *tm* nucleus medialis thalami; *tv* nucleus ventralis thalami; *tvm* nucleus ventralis medialis thalami

to that previously provided by physiological and pharmacological exploration of brain circuits involved in motor performance. Moreover, the changes in metabolic activity in some limbic areas may be of importance to the mental symptoms seen in Huntington's disease. This possibility argues for further more detailed exploration of these areas and their interconnections.

Acknowledgements

This work was supported by the W. Garfield Weston Foundation, the Huntington's Society of the United States and the Medical Research Council of Canada. Appreciation is extended to U. Scherer-Singler for excellent technical assistance.

References

Anderson, M., Yoshida, M.: Electrophysiological evidence for branching nigral projections to the thalamus and the superior collicus. Brain Research *137*, 361—364 (1977).

Burger, B., Thierry, A. M., Tassin, J. P., Moyne, M. A.: Dopaminergic innervation of the rat prefrontal cortex: A fluorescence histochemical study. Brain Research *106*, 133—145 (1976).

Coyle, J. T., McGeer, E. G., McGeer, P. L., Schwartz, R.: Neostriatal injections: A model for Huntington's chorea. In: Kainic Acid as a Tool in Neurobiology (*McGeer, E. G., Olney, J. W., McGeer, P. L.,* eds.), pp. 139—160. New York: Raven Press. 1978.

Fibiger, H. C.: Kainic acid lesions of the striatum: A pharmacological and behavioral model of Huntington's disease. In: Kainic Acid as a Tool in Neurobiology (*McGeer, E. G., Olney, J. W., McGeer, P. L.,* eds.), pp. 161—176. New York: Raven Press. 1978.

Gottesfeld, Z., Kvetnansky, R., Kopin, I. J., Jacobowitz, D. M.: Effects of repeated immobilization stress on glutamate decarboxylase and choline acetyltransferase in discrete brain regions. Brain Research *152*, 374—378 (1978).

Jakubovic, A., Lin, D., McGeer, E. G.: Protein and RNA synthesis in kainic acid-injected striata. Brain Research *163*, 289—294 (1979).

Kanazawa, I., Toyokura, Y.: Topographical study of the distribution of gamma-aminobutyric acid (GABA) in the human substantia nigra. A case study. Brain Research *100*, 371—381 (1975).

Kimura, H., Wada, J. A.: Metabolic exploration of amygdaloid (AM) kindled seizure using ^{14}C-2-deoxyglucose (DG) method. Am. Epil. Soc. Abstract, 1979.

König, J. F. R., Klippel, R. A.: The rat brain, a stereotaxic atlas of the forebrain and lower parts of the brain stem. Huntington, N.Y.: 1963.

McGeer, E. G., McGeer, P. L.: Some factors influencing the neurotoxicity of intrastriatal injections of kainic acid. Neurochem. Res. *3*, 501—517 (1978).

Nadler, J. V., Vaca, K. W., Frost White, W., Lynch, G. S., Cotman, C. W.: Aspartate and glutamate as possible transmitters of excitatory hippocampal afferents. Nature *260,* 538—540 (1976).

Schwartz, W. J., Sharp, F. R., Gunn, R. H., Evarts, E. V.: Lesions of ascending dopaminergic pathways decrease forebrain glucose uptake. Nature *261,* 155—157 (1976).

Sokoloff, L., Reivich, M., Kennedy, C., Des Rosiers, M. H., Patlak, C. S., Pettigrew, K. D., Sukurada, O., Shinohara, H.: The [^{14}C]deoxyglucose method for the measurement of local cerebral glucose utilization: theory procedure and normal values in the conscious and unconscious albino rat. J. Neurochem. *28,* 897—916 (1977).

Authors' address: Prof. *P. L. McGeer*, M.D., Laboratory of Neurological Research, University of British Columbia, 2075 Wesbrook Wall, Vancouver, B.C., Canada, V6T 1W5.

Journal of Neural Transmission, Suppl. 16, 111—128 (1980)
© by Springer-Verlag 1980

Progressive Supranuclear Palsy: Clinico-Pathological and Biochemical Studies

K. Jellinger, P. Riederer, and M. Tomonaga

Ludwig Boltzmann-Institute of Clinical Neurobiology, Lainz-Hospital, Wien, Austria, and Department of Clinical Pathology (Neuropathology), Tokyo Metropolitan Institute of Gerontology, Tokyo, Japan

With 5 Figures

Summary

Ten autopsy cases of Progressive Supranuclear Palsy (PSP) are reported. Age at onset ranged from 16 to 67 years and the duration of illness 3 to 24 years. The clinical features were aggressive mental retardation in 4 cases with early onset, paroxysmal dysequilibrium, ophthalmoplegia, rigidity and akinesia, pseudobulbar palsy and variable degrees of dementia. Neuropathology showed widespread neurofibrillary degeneration associated with system-bound neuronal loss and gliosis in subcortical areas, particularly affecting the subthalamic nucleus, substantia nigra, brainstem tegmentum and dentate nuclei, with no or little involvement of the cerebral cortex. The distribution of the lesions and the ultrastructure of the neurofibrillary tangles made of 15 nm straight filaments (seen in one case) in PSP are different from postencephalitic parkinsonism, Guam Parkinson-dementia complex and brainstem affection in (pre)senile dementia. Post-mortem biochemical analysis of two brains disclosed severe reduction of tyrosine hydroxylase, the key synthetic enzyme of the catecholamine pathway, not only in the nigro-striatal system as seen in Parkinson's disease, but in most areas of the brainstem and limbic system. The implication and possible pathogenic and therapeutic significance of these biochemical findings are discussed. The etiology of PSP and its nosological position within the degenerative extrapyramidal disorders remain unknown.

Introduction

Progressive supranuclear palsy (PSP) (*Steele et al.*, 1964), also referred to as Steele-Richardson-Olszewski syndrome (*Barbeau*, 1965)

and subcortical argyrophylic dystrophy (*Seitelberger*, 1969; *Jellinger*, 1971), is a progressive neurological disorder characterized by supra-nuclear opthalmoplegia, chiefly affecting vertical gaze (*Morax et al.*, 1974; *Mastaglia* and *Grainger*, 1975; *Troost* and *Daroff*, 1977), paroxysmal dysequilibrium, axial dystonia, rigidity, pseudobulbar palsy, mental impairment and less constant cerebellar and cortico-spinal signs. The pathological changes are widespread neurofibrillary degeneration, neuronal loss and gliosis in the brainstem, diencephalon and cerebellum with no or minimal cortical involvement. The remarkably constant clinical and pathological features and the ultra-structural appearance of the neurofibrillary tangles (NFT) in PSP, made of 15 nm straight filaments (*Tellez-Nagel* and *Wisniewski*, 1973; *Roy et al.*, 1974; *Powell et al.*, 1974; *Bugiani et al.*, 1979) have supported *Steele*'s (1972) contentation that the syndrome represents a distinct nosologic entity. However, the occurrence of 22 nm twisted tubules such as found in presenile and senile dementia, postencephalitic parkinsonism, Parkinson-Dementia complex, etc., have been described in one case (*Ishii* and *Ito*, 1979) and the presence of both straight and paired helical filaments has been observed in two cases (*Tomonaga*, 1977; *Probst*, 1977). Since transmission trials as yet have been un-successful (*Steele*, 1972), the etiology of this condition is unknown. Except for one case in which CSF studies suggested a defect in cerebral dopamine metabolism (*Mendell et al.*, 1970), no biochemical studies have been performed in PSP. Therapy has been unsatisfactory (*Albert et al.*, 1974; *Rouzaud et al.*, 1974; *Probst* and *Dufresne*, 1975; *Perkin et al.*, 1978) and only transient and moderate response of parkinsonian signs to L-dopa treatment (*Mendell et al.*, 1970) with no effect on the ocular disorders and dystonia has been reported (*Klawans* and *Ringel*, 1971).

This report presents the clinical and pathological findings in 10 cases of PSP, with electron microscopic studies in one, and bio-chemical analyses of post-mortem brains in two cases.

Clinical Data (Table 1)

There were 5 males and 5 females with an age range at death from 37 to 74 years, and a duration of the disease ranging from 3 to 24 years (mean 14.7 years). In no case was there any suggestion of familial incidence nor a history of previous encephalitis.

Two clinical types were observed.

(1) In four patients, all mentally subnormal, clinical symptoms began between 16 and 34 years of age with personality changes,

Table 1. *Major clinical symptoms in supranuclear palsy*

Case No.		1**	2	3	4*	5	6	7*	8	9	10
Age, sex		37 f	43 f	50 m	58 f	58 f	63 m	72 f	74 m	69 m	67 m
Age at onset (years)		8/16	20	26	37	43	58	67	57	60	64
Duration (years)		21	23	24	19	15	5	5	17	9	3
History of encephalitis		—	—	—	—	—	—	—	—	—	—
Initial symptoms	Mental retardation	++	++	++	+++	—	—	—	—	—	—
	Violent behavior	+++	+++	+++	+++	—	—	—	—	—	—
	Paroxysmal dysequilibrium	+	—	+	+	++	+	+	++	++	+++
	Unsteady gait	—	—	—	—	+	+	+	++	++	+++
	Defective convergence	++	—	—	+	—	+	+	—	++	+
	Altered vision	—	—	+	+	+	+	+	+	+	+
	Slurred speech	—	—	—	—	—	—	—	—	—	—
	Tremor	+	+	—	++	+	+	—	+	—	—
Fully developed disorder	Paroxysmal dysequilibrium	++	+	++	++	++	+++	++	+++	+++	+++
	Defective convergence	++	+	++	++	++	++	++	++	+++	+++
	Vert. gaze palsy	+++	+	+++	+++	+++	+++	++	+++	+++	+++
	Rigidity	+++	+	+++	++	++	+++	++	++	+++	+++
	Akinesia	+++	++	+++	++	+	++	++	+++	+++	+++
	Amimia, masked-face	+++	++	+++	++	++	++	++	++	+++	+++
	Sialorrhea	++	+	+	+	+	+	++	++	+++	++
	Dysarthria	—	—	—	—	—	—	—	—	++	++
	Dysphagia	+++	—	—	+	—	—	—	—	+	—
	Axial dystonia	—	—	—	+	—	—	+	+	+	—
	Tremor	++	—	—	—	—	—	—	+	+	+
	Hyperreflexia	—	—	—	+	+	+	+	—	—	—
	Pyramidal signs	—	—	—	—	—	—	—	+	—	—
	Pseudobulb. palsy	++	—	++	++	+	+	+	++	++	++
	Dementia	+	+	+	+	+	—	+	+	+	+
L-Dopa therapy effect		0	0	0	+—	+—	0	—	+	+—	—

— absent; +— minimal; + slight; ++ moderate; +++ severe; 0 not given.
* Reported by *Jellinger* (1971).
** Reported by *Seitelberger* (1969).

violent behaviour with outbursts of irritability and aggressiveness, restlessness and disorientation, causing early admission to psychiatric hospitals. Other initial signs were paroxysmal dysequilibrium with abrupt falls (2 cases), lid retraction or impaired convergence (2 patients), occasionally involuntary movements, *e.g.* mild generalized action tremor (case 1 and 4). In advanced stages of the disease, paroxysmal dysequilibrium with unsteady gait, defective convergence and vertical gaze palsy, progressive rigidity of the neck and limbs, amimia and mask-like face, bradykinesia, sialorrhea, dysarthria and dysphagia were present in cases 1, 3 and 4, and in two were associated with axial dystonia in extension. Complete ophthalmoplegia was present in case 4. Neither ophthalmoplegia nor pseudobulbar palsy were reported in case 2 who showed aggressive idiocy with outbursts of violence and mild rigidity, hypokinesia and dysarthria.

(2) The other six patients with later onset of symptoms at age 43 to 67 years initially presented with paroxysmal dysequilibrium, ataxic gait, speech and swallowing disorders, impairment of vision (diplopia) or defective convergence (3 cases), and progressive rigidity. Advanced clinical features became more stereotyped in all these patients, comprising widespread rigidity, mask-face and akinesia progressing to complete immobility, vertical gaze palsy or complete ophthalmoplegia (case 5, 6, 7, 10), and pseudobulbar palsy with dysarthria or anarthria and dysphagia (4 cases), tremor (2 cases) and unilateral or bilateral hyperreflexia with pyramidal signs (4 cases). Mild to moderate dementia was observed in 7 patients.

L-Dopa therapy performed in 6 patients, in three of which combined with L-deprenyl and/or bromocriptine induced a slight to moderate, but only transient improvement of rigidity and bradykinesia in 4 cases, with no favourable effect on ocular or behavioural disorders nor on the course of the disease. In two patients combined L-dopa treatment given in advanced phases induced no amelioration of symptoms at all. Laboratory data were unremarkable except for diffusely abnormal EEG records in advances stages of the disease and slight internal hydrocephalus on PEG or CT.

Neuropathology

Grossly, most brains showed mild diffuse cortical atrophy and internal hydrocephalus, the brain weights ranging from 1080 to 1480 g (mean 1253 g). Scars after bifrontal lobotomy were present in 2 cases, depigmentation of the substantia nigra was seen in 7 cases, three of which showed brownish pallido-nigral discoloration. The cerebellum and spinal cord (examined in 2 cases) showed nothing abnormal.

Histopathologically, slight atrophy and gliosis of the cerebral cortex was seen in all cases. Occasional senile plaques and NFT's in the neocortex were present in case 2 and 5, while small to moderate numbers of NFT's and a few senile plaques in the hippocampus were observed in 6 cases (case 2, 4, 5, 6, 7 and 8).

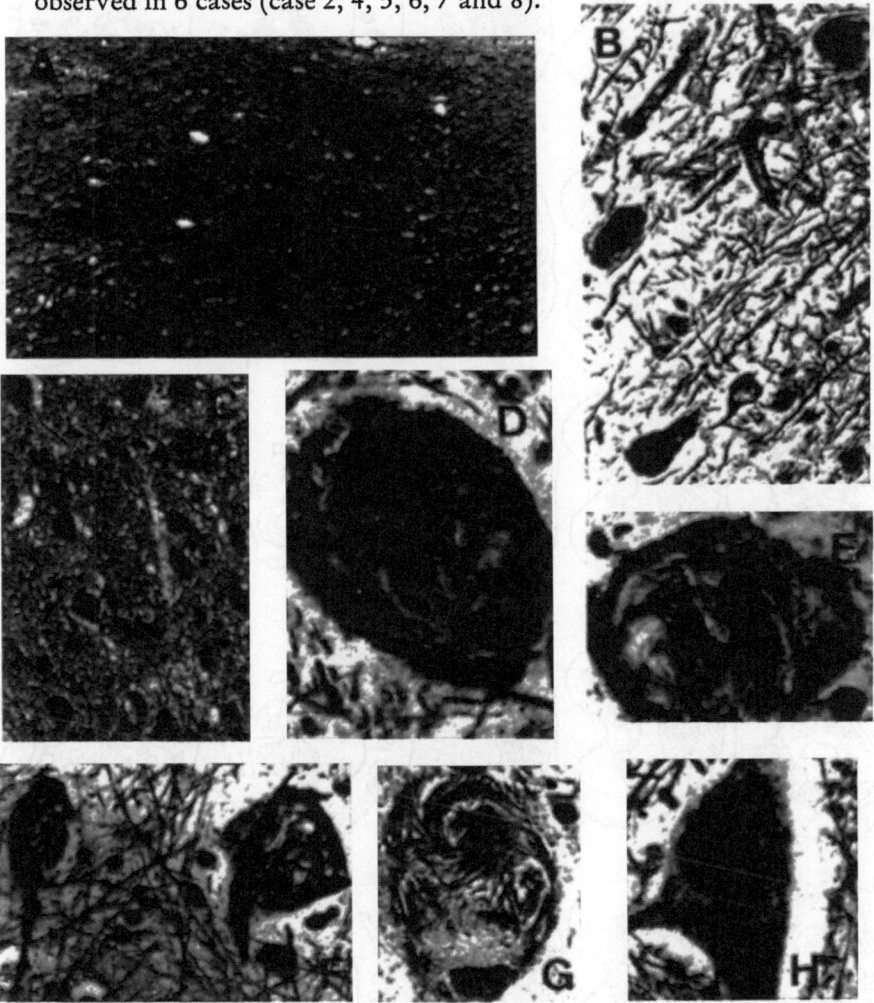

Fig. 1. *A* Neuronal loss and gliosis in subthalamic nucleus, H.E. ×60; *B* NFT in subthalamic nucleus, Bodian ×450; *C* Multiple NFT in nucleus centralis superior oralis, Bodian ×200; *D* Globose type of NFT in magnocellular reticular nucleus, Bodian ×1200; *E* Globose type of NFT in substantia nigra, Bodian ×1200; *F* Flame-shaped NFT in globus pallidus, Bodian ×600; *G* Globose type of NFT in oculomotor nucleus, K.V. ×800; *H* NFT in neuron from nucleus n. XII., Bodian ×800

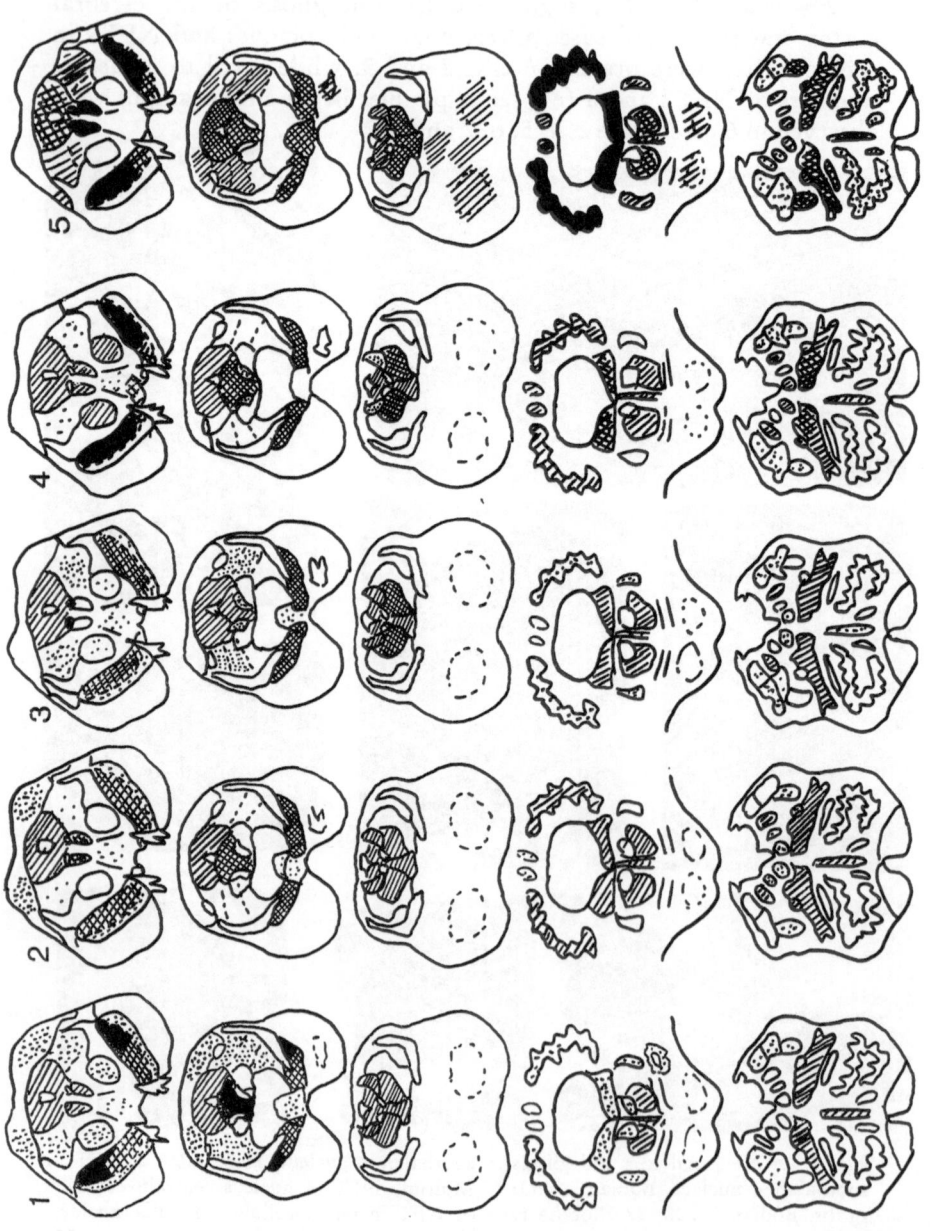

Fig. 2 (Legend see page 119)

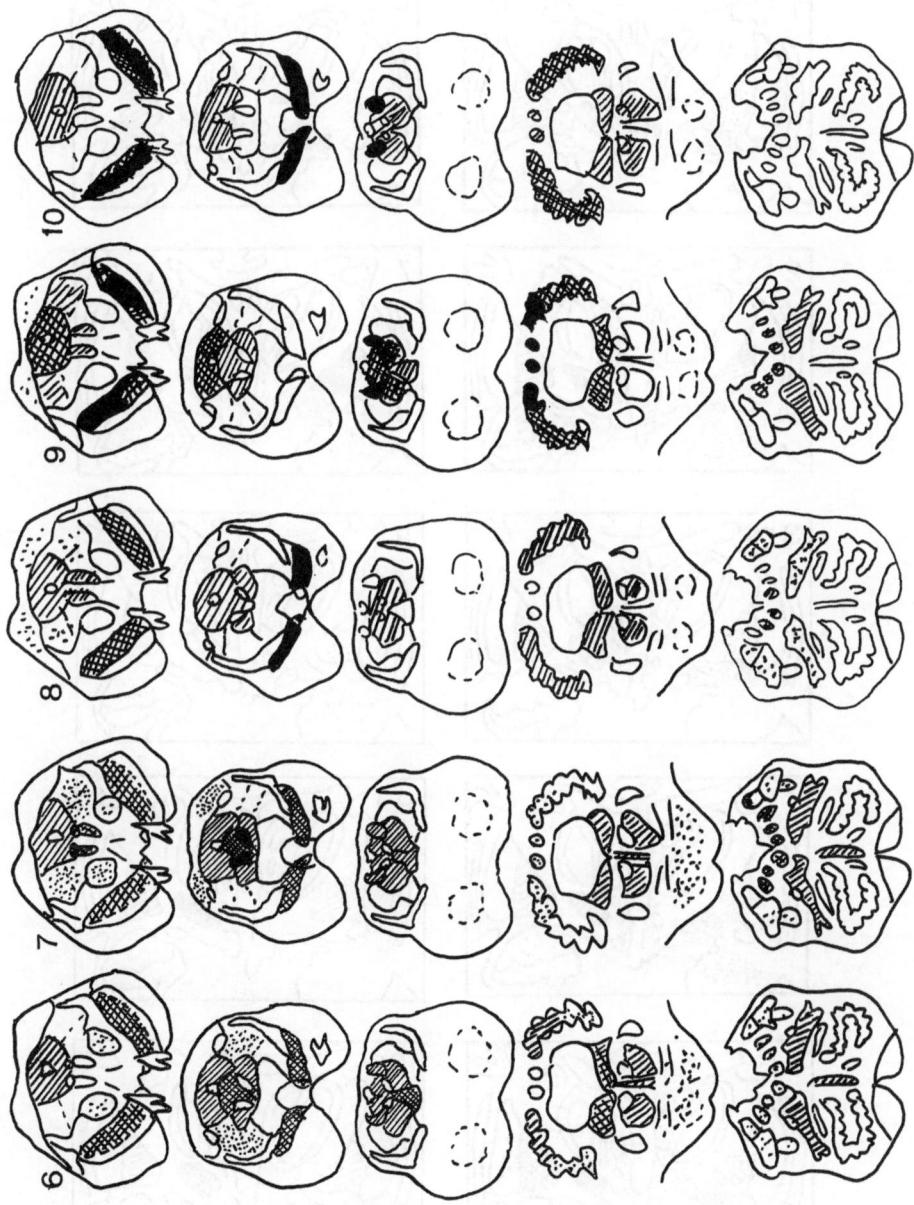

Fig. 2 (Legend see page 119)

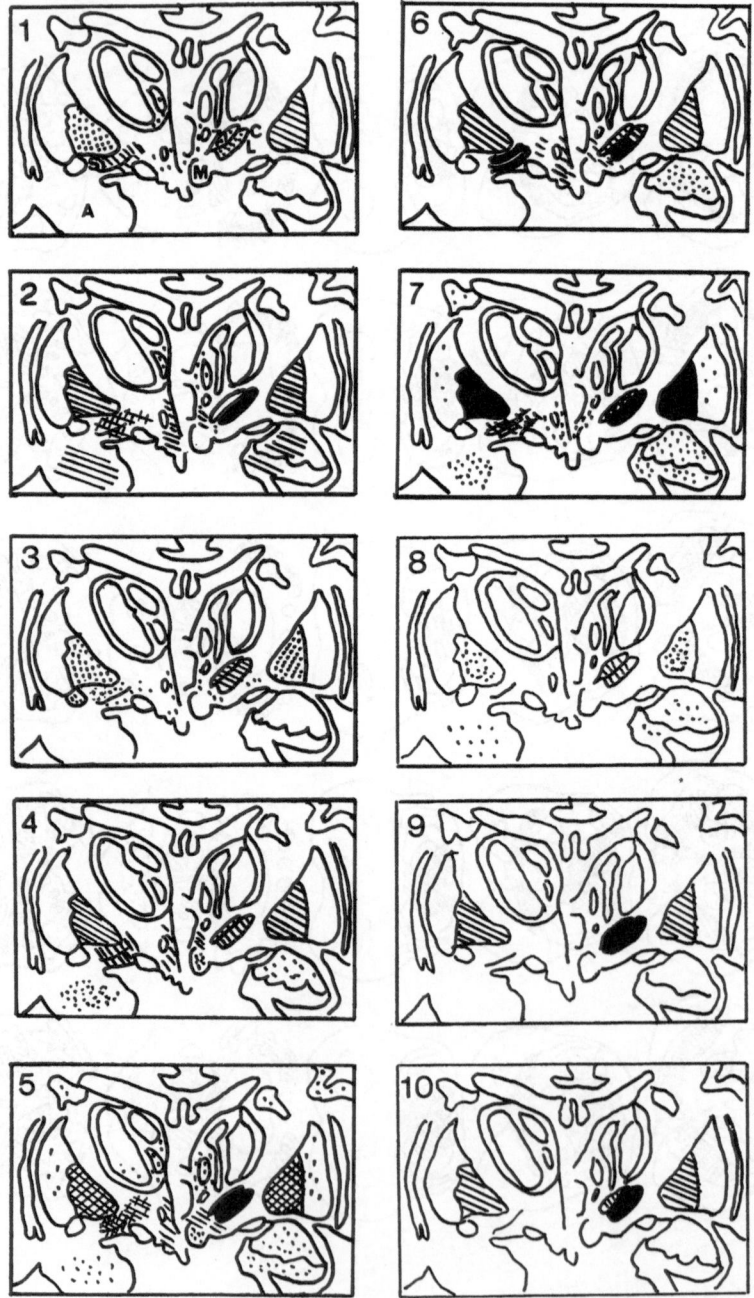

Fig. 3

There was abundance of neurofibrillary degeneration, moderate to severe neuronal loss, gliosis and occasional demyelination in various parts of the basal ganglia and brainstem. The NFT's occurring in the subcortical areas were both flame-shaped or globose in type (Figs. 1 B—H). The distribution of the lesions was remarkably constant except for the involvement of the dentate and pontine nuclei and the medulla oblongata. The pattern of the histopathological lesions evaluated semiquantitatively according to four degrees of severity is summarized in Figs. 2 and 3.

Almost constant sites of severe affection were the subthalamic nucleus and substantia nigra, less often the globus pallidus. Various degrees of neuronal loss, gliosis and occurrence of NFT's were associated with myelin pallor in globus pallidus, pallido-subthalamic tract, ansa lenticularis, and corpus subthalamicum, the latter often showing diffuse atrophy and gliosis with numerous NFT's (Figs. 1 A and B). Occasionally, increased amounts of iron and glial pigments with axonal spheroids were seen in the globus pallidus and reticular zone of substantia nigra, the latter showing no NFT's. There was severe involvement of the pars compacta of substantia nigra, with variable neuronal loss, depigmentation, gliosis and numerous NFT's. Sites of prominent affection were the ventromedial and dorsolateral oral nuclei and particularly the ventral, medial and dorsolateral nuclei of the caudal substantia nigra. Case 3 revealed only mild involvement of the oral part, the dorsal and lateral caudal nuclei, and moderate damage to the ventral and medial nuclei of the caudal substantia nigra. Abundance of NFT's with less severe degrees of neuronal loss and gliosis were seen in the pretectal region, tegmentum of the midbrain and pons including the periaqueductal gray matter, central superior pontine, locus coeruleus, oculomotor, trochlear, trigeminal, facial and abducens nuclei, substantia innominata, median raphé nuclei, magnocellular reticular (Fig. 1 D) and motor medullary nuclei, e.g. hypoglossus nuclei (Fig. 1 H). There was less severe and inconstant involvement of the posterior hypothalamus, dentate nuclei, corpora quadrigemina, pontine, cuneate and gracile nuclei. Occasional affection with scarce NFT's was present in the red nucleus, corpus

---

Figs. 2 and 3. Schematic pattern of lesions in 10 cases of PSP

⬚ Small number of NFT; little neuronal loss and gliosis

▨ Moderate number of NFT; moderate neuronal loss/gliosis

▩ Many NFT; moderate neuronal loss and gliosis

■ Many NFT; severe neuronal loss and gliosis (atrophy)

Table 2. *Biochemical studies in supranuclear palsy and Parkinson's disease*

	Tyrosine hydroxylase (nmol/g tissue/hour)			MAO (% inhibition)			
	Controls	Parkinson's disease	Supra-nuclear palsy 2543/78	Dopamine PSP Case 9	Parkinson's disease n = 3—7	Serotonin PSP Case 9	Parkinson's disease n = 3—7
Basal ganglia							
Caudate n.	27.8±2.3 (15)	3.5±1.0 (6)	0.7	—	89±2	—	64±12
Putamen	16.2±5.9 (5)	1.2±0.4 (6)	n.d.	—	88	—	38
Gl. pallidus	19.9±3.3 (3)	2.7±0.8 (4)	2.5	92/97	93±3	0	64±16
Diencephalon							
Thalamus	—	—	—	87/96	86±8	—	70±16
Hypothalamus	3.1±1.0 (5)	1.5±0.3 (3)	1.2	—	90	—	84
C. mamillare	—	—	—	92	94±3	9	58±22
Brainstem							
S. nigra	19.4±6.2 (4)	4.9±1.8 (4)	0.5	92/98	95±2	47/35	67±10
L. coeruleus	3.3±0.1 (4)	2.0±0.6 (2)	n.d.	92	95±2	19	67±17
N. ruber	5.7±1.9 (5)	2.1±1.4 (3)	n.d.	92/98	94±2	48/69	70±13
Raphé + F.R.	0.9±0.6 (4)	1.5±0.4 (5)	n.d.	—	93	—	83
Limbic system							
G. cinguli	—	—	—	92	93±6	20	65±19
N. amygdala	—	—	—	95	95±4	0	77±12
Hippocampus	—	—	—	92	94±3	30	66±24
G. dent.	—	—	—	93	94±2	10	65±25
N. accumbens	2.0±0.7 (5)	2.7±1.2 (9)	1.2	92	93±3	0	65±12
Dendate n.	—	—	—	91	—	—	—
Frontal cortex	—	—	—	92	94±2	0	60±20

n.d. = not detectable; number of patients in parenthesis; x ± S.E.M.; — = not determined.

striatum, thalamus and inferior olives, while the cerebellar cortex was preserved. Lewy bodies in substantia nigra and/or locus coeruleus were seen in two cases. The *spinal cord* examined in two cases showed mild neuronal loss with occasional NFT's in the intermediate gray matter of one, without damage to the spinal tracts and nerve roots.

Electron Microscopy

Small blocks of formalin-fixed material of substantia nigra and pontine superior central nucleus were post-fixed in glutaraldehyde and osmium-tetroxide, processed for electron microscopy, and observed with a JEM 100B microscope.

The NFT's were composed of clusters of straight filaments, commonly arranged in circling and interlacing bundles (Fig. 4). The filaments were of indeterminate lenght and measured 12—20 nm in width, with an average diameter of 15 nm and their central region was seldom electron lucent. Occasional narrowings to 9—11 nm without evidence of periodicity were present, but no paired helical filaments were observed in the material examined.

Biochemistry (Table 2)

Post-mortem brain tissue were obtained from 2 patients (case 8 and 9) 3 and 7 hours after death, respectively. Tyrosine hydroxylase (TH) activity was measured radioenzymatically using the method of *McGeer et al.* (1967). The results were compared to age-matched controls and cases of Parkinson's disease (see *Birkmayer et al.*, 1974; *Riederer* and *Wuketich*, 1976; *Riederer et al.*, 1978).

TH, the key synthetic enzyme of the catecholamine pathway, was most severely reduced in the nigrostriatal system and no activity was detected in several brainstem nuclei. Except for the globus pallidus, TH reduction in PSP was found to be more pronounced than in Parkinson's disease.

The inhibition of dopamine monoaminoxidase (MAO) by (—)deprenyl examined in case 9 was similar when compared to a group of 3—7 brains of Parkinson's disease. However, when using 5-HT as substrate, the inhibition was considerably lower than in Parkinson's disease. In parkinsonian patients the last administration of (—)deprenyl given 10 mg per day had been 5 to 35 hours before death, while in case 9 of PSP the drug was given 48 hours before death. If this lower inhibition is not a PSP-specific finding, it is suggested that the inhibition of 5-HT-MAO disappears more rapidly than the blockade of dopamine-MAO.

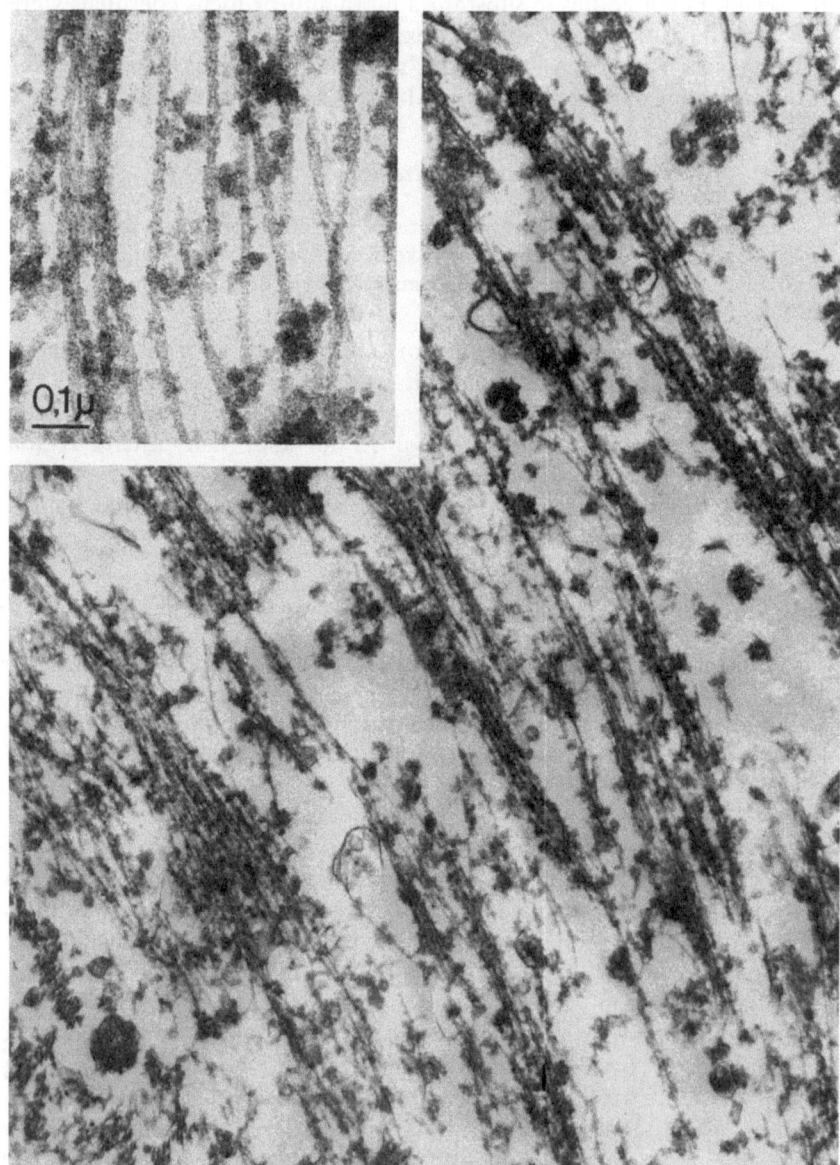

Fig. 4. Part of NFT observed in the superior central pontine nucleus, consisting of parallel and interlacing bundles of straight tubules. ×36,000. Inset: Detail of the straight filaments showing well-defined borders with superimposed electrondense granular cytoplasmic material. ×120,000

Discussion

The clinical syndrome of PSP which may take many years to develop fully, comprises (supra)nuclear ophthalmoplegia, pseudobulbar palsy, axial dystonia, rigidity, akinesia and mental disturbances. Symptoms most often begin in the fifth and sixth decade with unsteady gait, altered vision, changes in personality and difficulty in speech and swallowing (*Steele*, 1972), while earlier onset in mentally retarded young adults with violent behaviour and involuntary movements observed in 4 of our patients appears to be rare (*Colmant*, 1971; *Seitelberger*, 1969). Supra- or internuclear ophthalmoplegia, particularly for vertical gate, the hallmark of the disease (*Mastaglia* and *Grainger*, 1975; *Troost* and *Daroff*, 1977; *Perkin et al.*, 1978), has been present in all reported cases except our case 2, but may be inconspicuous in the early stages of the condition (*Kurihara et al.*, 1974; *Morax et al.*, 1974; *Perkin et al.*, 1978). Although unusual, there may be mild degree of tremor at rest or action tremor (*Barbeau*, 1965; *Probst* and *Dufresne*, 1975). Intellectual dysfunction, a frequent but inconsistent feature of PSP, is characterized by forgetfulness, slowing of thought process, emotional and behavioral changes with outbursts of violence and aggressiveness (*Steele et al.*, 1964; *Ishino et al.*, 1975). These behavior changes which may resemble the dementia occurring after bifrontal lobe disease, have been referred to as "subcortical dementia" (*Albert et al.*, 1974) or "pseudodementia" (*Constantinidis et al.*, 1970). In the later stages, progressive rigidity and akinesia with masked face and pseudobulbar palsy with dysphagia and anarthria reduce the patient to a helpless bedridden state and death supervenes in two to 24 years. The advanced clinical picture is reminiscent of akinetic parkinsonism and, although the association of ophthalmoplegia and bulbar palsy militates against such a diagnosis (*Steele*, 1972) and the eye movement disorders in postencephalitis parkinsonism are not comparable with those in PSP (*Troost* and *Daroff*, 1977; *Perkin et al.*, 1978), many cases of PSP clinically have been considered as some type of parkinsonism (*Steele*, 1972; *Bugiani et al.*, 1979).

The association of widespread neurofibrillary degeneration and systemic neuronal loss and gliosis in subcortical areas, with little or no cortical involvement, the pathological hallmark of PSP, is also seen in a variety of conditions, *e.g.* postencephalitic parkinsonism and Guam P-D-complex, which, however, show different patterns of lesion (*Hirano et al.*, 1966; *Ishino et al.*, 1975). In presenile and senile dementia, cortical involvement is accompanied by inconstant occurrence of NFT's in various brainstem areas, the distribution of which, however, differs from that in PSP (*Jellinger*, 1971; *Ishino et al.*, 1975). Semiquantitative evaluation of the brainstem lesions in 90 demented persons aged 55 to 92 years (average 75 years) showed the following distribution in descending order of frequency and intensity (Fig. 5): n. supratrochlearis, n. centralis pontis oralis, n. dorsalis raphé, locus coeruleus, n. magnocellularis reticularis, n. interpeduncularis, zona compacta nigrae, zona incerta, posterior hypothalamus and n. subcuneiformis, while the globus pallidus, subthalamic nucleus, thalamus, oculomotor dentate and medullary motor nuclei were rarely affected. By contrast, occurrence of senile plaques in the limbic system and inferior nuclei is not the feature of PSP. Furthermore, there are differences in the ultrastructure of subcortical NFT's observed in different conditions. While NFT's occurring in senile and presenile dementia, postencephalitic parkinsonism, Guam P-D-complex and other chronic diseases are known to belong to the paired helical filament type (*Wisniewski* and *Soffer*, 1979), the NFT's in PSP show a unique pattern of 15 nm straight filaments, either in isolation (*Tellez-Nagel* and *Wisniewski*, 1973; *Roy et al.*, 1974; *Powell et al.*, 1974; *Bugiani et al.*, 1969) or in association with paired helical filaments (*Tomonaga*, 1977; *Probst*, 1977). Both types

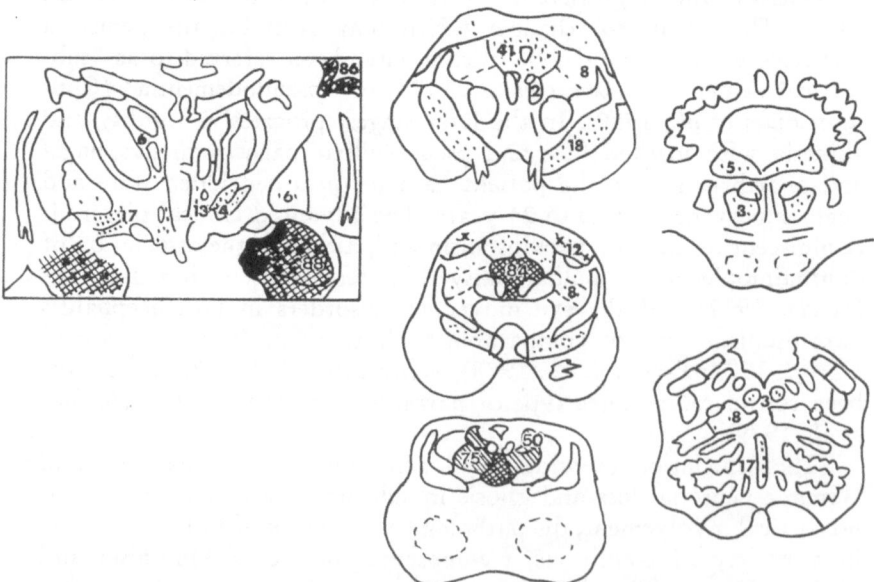

Fig. 5. Incidence of NFT's and senile plaques in 90 unselected brains of aged persons (average 75 years) with presenile and senile dementia. Numbers indicate positive findings; severity of NFT's is given in four degrees: ■■■ severe, ▨▨▨ moderate, ▨▨▨ slight, ⌐⋯⋯⌐ very slight (singular)

were observed separately in each brainstem neuron, but only a few straight filaments were mixed with the paired helical filaments in occasional cortical tangles (*Yagishita et al.*, 1979). Although no transition between these two structures was observed, their distribution and concurrence suggest that (a) the same neurons are capable of assembling different types of fibrillary material in various pathological conditions which, (b) in their origin may be related to each other, although the underlying disorders of neuronal protein metabolism are still unknown. It remains undetermined, whether PSP represents a particular type of "subcortical argyrophilic dystrophy" with ensuing systemic degeneration of the affected neuronal pathways, or a primary heterogenous system degeneration with a particular pattern of lesions and of neurofibrillary degeneration.

The broad clinical spectrum of PSP which is that of a slowly progressive extrapyramidal disorder resembling akinetic parkinsonism associated with ophthalmoplegia, pseudobulbar palsy and behavioral changes is considered to be related to the pattern of subcortical pathology affecting various neuronal and neurotransmitter systems. Ophthalmoplegia and pseudobulbar palsy correlate well with distinctive location of pathological changes to nuclei of the brainstem tegmentum. Akinesia and other "parkinsonian" symptoms in PSP can be related to the consistantly severe involvement of the substantia nigra and degeneration of the dopaminergic nigrostriatal pathway documented by our biochemical data. In both Parkinson's disease and PSP there is a significant reduction of tyrosine hydroxylase, the key synthetic enzyme of the catecholamine pathway, in the striatum, diencephalon and limbic structures, although there is a different behavior of this enzyme in various brain areas between parkinsonism (*Lloyd et al.*, 1975; *McGeer et al.*, 1976; *Nagatsu et al.*, 1977; *Riederer et al.*, 1978) and PSP. While in Parkinson's disease the loss of TH activity particularly affects the nigrostriatal system with only little involvement of other areas of the brainstem and limbic system (*Riederer et al.*, 1978), PSP shows a significant loss of TH activity in almost all brainstem areas and some limbic structures, indicating a widespread degeneration of presynaptic dopaminergic neurons. Moreover, preliminary data show that spiroperon binding, which is thought to act on postsynaptic dopaminergic neurons is much more decreased in one case of PSP than in Parkinson's disease (*Owen et al.*, 1980). In addition, ADTN-binding in PSP is reduced below the levels observed in Parkinson's disease. Both types of binding are also severely affected in the n. accumbens, a mesolimbic area. Hence, in PSP there is apparently a much more severe and widespread degeneration of subcortical dopaminergic pathways than in par-

kinsonian syndromes, affecting not only the nigrostriatal dopaminergic fibers, but also other neurons of the brainstem and mesolimbic
system.

These changes may also be of importance for the frequent
behavioral changes with emotional irritability and "subcortical
dementia" which have been related to degeneration of the brainstem
reticular formation (*Ishino et al.*, 1975) and of the mesolimbic and
mesocortical limbic dopaminergic systems that are considered to
represent an anatomical basis for the self-stimulating behavioral
disorders (*Stevens* and *Livermore*, 1978). In parkinsonism, mental
symptoms including psychotic phases also appear to be localized in
extrastriatal areas (*Birkmayer* and *Riederer*, 1975). The preliminary
results of our biochemical studies may also explain the conflicting
results of L-dopa treatment in PSP inducing transient improvement
of "parkinsonian" symptoms, without significant effects on other
clinical symptoms, but further attempts to correlate clinico-
therapeutic experiments and neuropathological data with neurochemical assays of the regional cerebral transmitter metabolism will
be warranted in order to elucidate the pathophysiological problems
of this disorder.

References

Albert, M. L., Feldman, R. G., Willis, A. L.: "The subcortical dementia" of
progressive supranuclear palsy. J. Neurol. Neurosurg. Psychiat. *37*,
121—130 (1974).

Barbeau, A.: Dégénérescence plurissystématisée du névrauxe. Syndrome de
Steele-Richardson-Olszewski. Un. méd. Canada *94*, 715—718 (1965).

Birkmayer, W., Danielczyk, W., Neumayer, E., Riederer, P.: Nucleus ruber
and L-Dopa psychosis. Biochemical post-mortem findings. J. Neural
Transm. *35*, 93—116 (1974).

Birkmayer, W., Riederer, P.: Responsibility of extrastriatal areas for the
appearance of psychotic symptoms. J. Neural Transm. *37*, 175—182
(1975).

Bugiani, L., Mancardi, G. L., Brusa, A., Ederli, E.: The fine structure of subcortical neurofibrillary tangles in progressive supranuclear palsy. Acta
Neuropath. (Berlin) *45*, 147—152 (1979).

Colmant, H. J.: Progressive supranuclear palsy. Arch. Psychiat. Nervenkr.
214, 324—330 (1971).

Constantinidis, J., Tissot, R., De Ajuriaguerra, J.: Dystonie oculo-facio-
cervicale ou paralysie progressive supranucléaire de Steele-Richardson-
Olszewski. Rev. neurol. *122*, 249—262 (1970).

Hirano, A., Malamud, N., Elizan, T. S., Kurland, L. T.: Amyotrophic lateral
sclerosis and Parkinson-dementia complex on Guam. Arch. Neurol.
(Chic.) *15*, 35—51 (1966).

Ishii, Y., Itoh, T.: An autopsy case of progressive supranuclear palsy. Clin. Neurol. (Tokyo) *19*, 187 (1979).

Ishino, H., Ikeda, H., Otsuki, S.: Contribution to the clinical pathology of progressive supranuclear palsy (subcortical argyrophilic dystrophy). J. Neurol. Sci. *24*, 471—481 (1975).

Jellinger, K.: Progressive supranuclear palsy (subcortical argyrophilic dystrophy). Acta Neuropath. (Berlin) *19*, 347—352 (1971).

Klawans, H. L., Ringel, S. P.: Observations on the efficacy of L-Dopa in progressive supranuclear palsy. Europ. Neurol. *5*, 115—129 (1975).

Kurihara, T., Landau, W. M., Torack, R. M.: Progressive supranuclear palsy with actions myoclonus, seizures. Neurology (Minneap.) *24*, 219—223 (1971).

Mastaglia, F. L., Grainger, K. M. R.: Internuclear opthalmoplegia in progressive supranuclear palsy. J. Neurol. Sci. *25*, 303—308 (1975).

McGeer, E. G., Gibson, S., McGeer, P. L.: Some characteristics of brain tyrosine hydroxylase. Canad. J. Biochem. *45*, 1557—1563 (1967).

McGeer, P. L., Hattori, T., Singh, V. K., McGeer, E. G.: Cholinergic symptoms on extrapyramidal function. In: Basal Ganglia (*Ahr, M. D.,* ed.), pp. 213—222. New York: Plenum Press. 1976.

Mendell, J. R., Chase, T. N., Engel, W. K.: Modification by L-Dopa of a case of progressive supranuclear palsy. With evidence of defective cerebral dopamine metabolism. Lancet *I*, 593—594 (1970).

Morax, P. U., Aron-Rosa, D., Barthold, I., Contamin, F., Mignot, M.: Les paralysies supranucléaires progressives. Ann. Oculist (Paris) *207*, 267 to 278 (1974).

Nagatsu, T., Kato, T., Numata, Y., Ikuta, K., Sano, M., et al.: Phenyl-ethanolamine-N-methyl transferase and other enzymes of catecholamine metabolism in human brain. Clin. Chim. Acta *75*, 221—232 (1977).

Owen, F., Cross, A. J., Crow, T. J., Reynolds, G., Riederer, P.: In preparation.

Perkin, G. D., Lees, A. J., Stern, G. M., Kolen, R. S.: Problems in the diagnosis of progressive supranuclear palsy (Steele-Richardson-Olszewski Syndrome). Canad. J. Neurol. Sci. *5*, 167—173 (1978).

Powell, H. C., London, G. W., Lampert, P. W.: Neurofibrillary tangles in progressive supranuclear palsy. Electron microscopic observations. J. Neuropath. exp. Neurol. *33*, 98—106 (1974).

Probst, A.: Dégénérescence de neurofibrillaire sous-corticale senile avec presence de tubule contournés et de filaments droits. Forme atypique de la paralysie supranucléaire progressive. Rev. Neurol. *133*, 417—428 (1977).

Probst, A., Dufresne, J. J.: Paralysie supranucléaire progressive ou dystonie oculo-facio-cervicale. Arch. Suisses Neurol. Neurochir. Psychiat. *116*, 107—134 (1975).

Riederer, P., Rausch, W. D., Birkmayer, W., Jellinger, K., Seemann, D.: CNS modulation of adrenal tyrosine hydroxylase in Parkinson's disease and metabolic encephalopathies. J. Neural Transm., Suppl. 14, 121—131. Wien-New York: Springer. 1978.

Riederer, P., Wuketich, S.: Time course of nigrostriatal degeneration in Parkinson's disease. J. Neural Transm. *38*, 277—301 (1976).

Rouzaud, M., Degiovanni, E., Jobard, P., Gray, E., Durand, J. P.: L'ophthalmoplegie supranucléaire progressive (Syndrome de Steele-Richardson-Olszewski). Rev. Neurol. *130*, 143—164 (1974).

Roy, S., Datta, C. K., Hirano, A., Ghatak, N. R., Zimmerman, H. M.: Electron microscopic study of neurofibrillary tangles in Steele-Richardson-Olszewski syndrome. Acta Neuropath. (Berlin) *29*, 175 to 179 (1974).

Seitelberger, F.: Heterogenous system degeneration. Subcortical argyrophilic dystrophy. Acta Neurol. (Napoli) *24*, 276—284 (1969).

Steele, J. C.: Progressive supranuclear palsy. Brain *95*, 693—704 (1972).

Steele, J. C., Richardson, J. C., Olszewski, J.: Progressive supranuclear palsy. Arch. Neurol. (Chic.) *10*, 333—359 (1964).

Stevens, J. R., Livermore, A., jr.: Kindling of the mesolimbic dopamine system: Animal model of psychosis. Neurology (Minneap.) *28*, 36—46 (1978).

Tellez-Nagel, I., Wisniewski, H. M.: Ultrastructure of neurofibrillary tangles in Steele-Richardson-Olszewski syndrome. Arch. Neurol. (Chic.) *29*, 324—327 (1973).

Tomonaga, M.: Ultrastructure of neurofibrillary tangles in progressive supranuclear palsy. Acta Neuropath. (Berlin) *37*, 177—181 (1977).

Troost, B. T., Daroff, R. B.: The ocular motor defects in progressive supranuclear palsy. Ann. Neurol. *2*, 397—403 (1977).

Yagishita, S., Itoh, Y., Amano, N., Nakano, T., Saitoh, A.: Ultrastructure of neurofibrillary tangles in progressive supranuclear palsy. Acta Neuropath. (Berlin) *48*, 27—30 (1979).

Wisniewski, H. M., Soffer, D.: Neurofibrillary pathology: current status and research perspectives. Mech. Ageing Developm. *9*, 119—142 (1979).

Authors' address: Prof. Dr. *K. Jellinger,* Ludwig Boltzmann-Institute of Clinical Neurobiology, Lainz-Hospital, Wolkersbergenstrasse 1, A-1130 Wien, Austria.

Journal of Neural Transmission, Suppl. 16, 129—136 (1980)

Clinical Analysis of Akinesia

H. Narabayashi

Department of Neurology, Juntendo Medical School, Tokyo, Japan

With 2 Figures

Summary

Symptoms called akinesia in movement are analysed and classified into three groups. The first is that secondary to existence of marked rigidity of muscles and the second is that due to striatal dopamine deficiency, which simply be interpreted as "lack of movement". The third is freezing or festination in quick repetitive movement especially in gait, speech and handwriting, for which l-Dopa therapy has no influence. Specific difficulty in the latter condition is found in the rhythm formation of repetitive movements when repetition is over 2 Hz, which the author named "hastening phenomenon converging into 5 Hz".

However, the neural mechanism and pathology under the third group of akinesia is still not known. In most of the parkinsonian patients, it is considered that all three groups of akinesia are mixed together with variety of grade. Careful observations on the changes of clinical pictures through the course of l-Dopa therapy and of stereotaxic surgery provided the analysis of so-called akinesia as described.

Development and success of pharmacological treatment for parkinsonism, which was pioneered by Viennese group of scientists around Prof. Birkmayer, introduced the enthusiasm in neuropharmacology and transmitter research in one hand, but also it offered many interesting aspects of clinical investigation on this disease. Akinesia is one of the main topics.

Today, rigidity, tremor and akinesia are recognized well as the three axial motor symptoms of the disease. However, the clear and very recognition of akinesia belongs to relatively recent knowledge and was first established by the observation that the symptom of akinesia remains still after complete elimination of rigidity by stereo-taxic surgery. Before that the term akinesia itself had not been the clear defined term and often mixed with motor-difficulty caused by rigidity.

This paper aims to analyse and interpret the various clinical symptoms called akinesia of wide sense into three groups by objective devices.

Clinical descriptions of akinesia include the wide variety of motor symptoms, such as poverty of facial mimic, loss of blinking, low voice, dysarthria, and decrease or slowness of movements in general, such as decrease or diminution of arm swinging during walk, marche petit pas or difficulty in quick repetitive movement. Also the peculiar symptom called freezing or festination, which is often described as difficulty in initiation or start of movement, is included within the frame of akinetic symptoms [5].

These varieties of symptoms may not be uniform in their mechanisms of generation and may be caused by several different neural mechanisms, which interfere with human motor performance.

1. First Group of Akinetic Symptoms

Some of the akinetic symptoms can be produced secondarily by existence of marked rigidity of muscles. For example, existence of rigidity on both extensor and flexor muscles of extremity produces disturbance of reciprocal inhibition. Elimination of muscular rigidity on the extremities contralateral to the stereotaxic thalamotomy in a case of hemiparkinsonism, produces normalization in the skill and speed of repetitive movements such as finger opening and first making, supination and pronation movement of the forearm, of arm swinging, of facial mimic and of elevation of heel during walking or stepping. This is the clear proof that the difficulties in these movements are secondarily caused by existence of rigidity of muscles, which is diffuse and nonreciprocal in nature on all skeletal muscles of the affected extremity [10]. Such improvement by surgery is best obtained in the unilaterally affected case than in the bilateral severe case. Detailed neurophysiological investigation about the mechanism of rigidity or of tremor generation may not be described in this paper and better be referred to other papers by the author [9].

Fig. 1 is an example of wrist movement in a case of 52 year-old male patient with hemiparkinsonism of the left side and of six years duration. Muscle activity is described by surface electromyography through bipolar plate electrodes placed on the muscle belly. In the

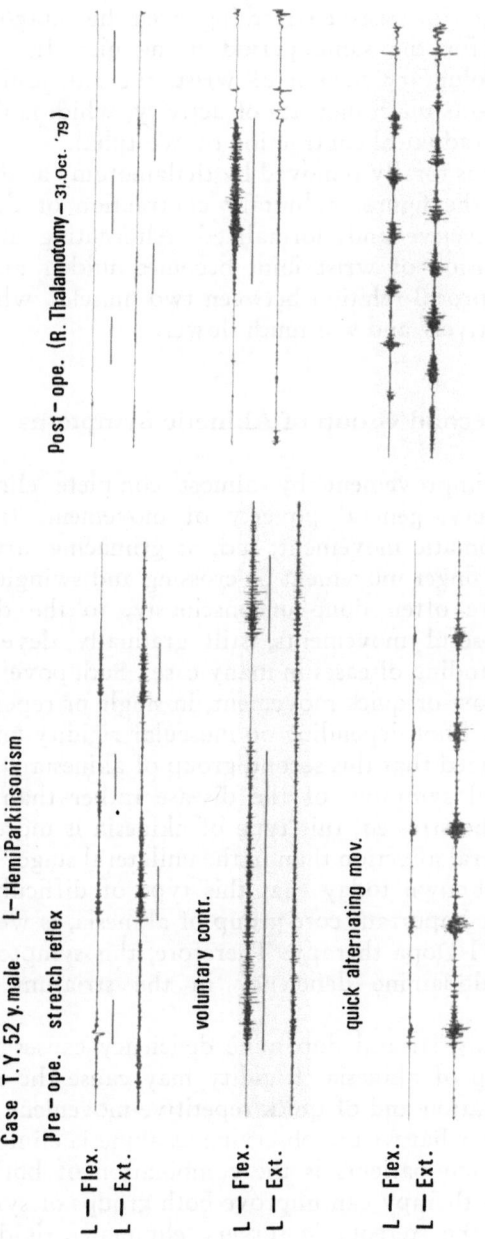

Fig. 1. Disturbance of reciprocity in movement in rigid parkinsonian extremity (see the text): *Flex.* forearm flexor muscle, *Ext.* forearm extensor muscle

preoperative rigid state, which is manifested by existence of tonic muscular discharges for passive stretching, even the antagonist showed tonic discharges for the same period as agonist. In a chance of carefully done voluntary flexion of wrist, the antagonist (extensor muscle) also presents much increase of activity, which is the phenomenon named as paradoxical contraction by Westphal.

When rigidity is totally removed by thalamotomy as shown on the right column in the figure, voluntary contraction of flexor muscle becomes more selective and normalized. Alternating movement of flexion and extension of wrist joint becomes quicker and smoother with normal reciprocal relation between two muscles, which was not possible preoperatively and was much slower.

2. Second Group of Akinetic Symptoms

In spite of improvement by almost complete elimination of rigidity by surgery, general poverty of movement, from loss of delicate and automatic movement, such as grimacing, arm swinging, delicate arm and finger movement or crossing and swinging of legs in sitting, which are often done unconsciously, to the difficulty of voluntary purposeful movements, still gradually develops in the course of long-standing diseases in many cases. Such poverty of movement, either in slow or quick movement, in single or repetitive movement, is considered not depending on muscular rigidity and it became gradually recognized that this second group of akinesia was definitely the most essential symptom of the disease rather than rigidity or tremor. It must be stressed, this type of akinesia is more marked in the stage of bilateral affection than in the unilateral stage.

It is widely known today that this type of difficulty, which is actually the most important core group of akinesia, is well improved and modified by l-Dopa therapy. Therefore, this symptom is one of the results of dopamine deficiency in the striatum as well as rigidity [1, 2].

In other words, striatal dopamine deficiency causes rigidity and this second group of akinesia. Rigidity may cause the difficulty of reciprocal innervation and of quick repetitive movement as described above. Therefore, what we are observing as akinesia clinically in most of the parkinsonian patients is the combination of both groups of akinesia. L-Dopa therapy can improve both groups of symptoms. On the other hand, the stereotaxic surgery eliminates rigidity and the rigidity depending hypokinesia or bradykinesia only, but does not influence at all the second group of akinesia.

Another important observation is that the second group of akinetic symptoms which gradually develops within several years even after the successful surgery on rigidity, unilaterally or bilaterally, respond well to the l-Dopa therapy afterwards, as in the cases which had no surgery. When l-Dopa therapy was introduced widely to the practice around 1960, many cases which underwent surgery several months or years ago received l-Dopa therapy with the similarly good response to this new drug as in the non-operated cases. This was also described by *Hughes et al.* (1971) [3]. Such observation may suggest that the neural mechanism of producing the second group of akinesia may not be via the pallido-thalamic pathway, which was already blocked exactly by the stereotaxic lesion of a few millimeter diameter either in the internal pallidum or in the ventrolateral nucleus of the thalamus. In contrast, rigidity producing mechanism is conveyed by this projection. For the second group of akinesia, therefore, another neural pathways must be postulated and the real neural mechanism of producing this type of akinesia and also of improving this symptom by drugs are still not clearly explained at all.

3. Third Group of Akinetic Symptoms

With increase of experiences in l-Dopa therapy for about ten years, interesting observations or new understanding of symptoms in this disease are gradually accumulated, which were not well defined previously. One of those symptoms better recognized through long-term l-Dopa therapy is the third group of akinetic symptoms, which is named as the freezing phenomenon or the difficulty of initiation or of start of movement.

Patients presenting this symptom can paradoxically step up or down the staircase almost normally, although the walking on the floor or through the door or the narrow gate is severely disturbed by appearance of gait freezing. He also paradoxically can step over the obstacle on the floor, even when his gait is frozen.

Freezing or a similar phenomenon called festination has been known as a symptom frequently seen in parkinsonism, but was not established as an independent symptom from rigidity and tremor or as different from the former two groups of akinetic symptoms.

In some selected cases of parkinsonism, in which the long-term l-Dopa therapy is successfully applied for more than five or six years and the gratifying results of almost complete diminution of rigidity and akinesia with normalized ADL is obtained, slight tendency of freezing phenomenon starts to appear, which is often slowly progressive and finally makes the patients unable to walk. The patients with this difficulty often present the similar difficulty in handwriting and speech parallely. However, the difficulty is mainly for start or performance of ordinary or rapid repetitive movements and the movements of slow tempo can easily and steadily be performed. There exist no noticeable rigidity, tremor or weakness of muscles, because of the pharmacological and in some cases of previous neurosurgical treatment. Further increase in the dosage of l-Dopa usually does not lessen the difficulty but often tends to worsen it. This difficulty is different from the second group of akinetic symptoms in that the patient can perform the slow repetitive movements almost normally and steadily, although for the patients with the second group of akinesia movements of any tempo, either slow or quick, are almost impossible.

The author with Nakamura tried to analyse the mechanism of this peculiar type of akinesia, *i.e.* the freezing phenomenon, by simple clinical device, which was described elsewhere in detail and therefore will be referred briefly [4, 6, 7].

The finger-tapping test with the small mental plate in the middle finger is used. The plate may touch another metal plate on the table, thus closing the circuit to be registered electrically. When the patient is asked to make tapping freely with maximum speed, the upper limit of repetition of tapping is usually around 5—6 Hz, which seems close to tremor frequency, though the normal age-matched control subjects would be able to perform by around 8—9 Hz.

When the tapping in response to the given photic or sonic signal of varied frequency is requested, these patients can follow the signal well until the frequency of 2 Hz. When the frequency goes over 2 Hz, the patient cannot follow exactly, get confused and his tapping rate automatically converges into the frequency of around 5 Hz almost always, which is the phenomenon named by us as "hastening phenomenon", though the normal control subjects can still follow the signal frequency until 7 or 8 Hz (Fig. 2).

From these simple analysis, it is suggested that the parkinsonian patients have the specific difficulty to perform the repetitive alternative movements in the frequency other than 5 Hz, except when the frequency is low as below 2 Hz. Table 1 summarizingly indicates such peculiar feature of rhythmic movements in the disease. *Wertham* (1929) has first described such difficulty in rhythmic movements as "arrhythmokinesia" [11].

We also have demonstrated that such disturbance of rhythm formation in parkinsonism is an independent symptom from rigidity and tremor. It is also different from the second category of akinetic symptoms in that the patient can perform the delicate repetitive movements under the frequency of 2 Hz, though the latter has difficulty in performing the movement under any frequency, even below 2 Hz.

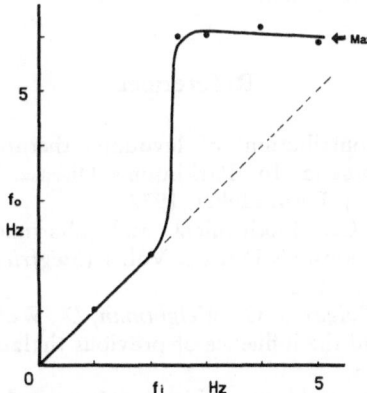

Fig. 2. Typical course of freezing in responsive tapping in a case of parkinsonism for different frequency signals. When the given signal (*fi*) is below 2 Hz, tapping (*f$_o$*) is of the same frequency, but when over 2.5 Hz, the response (*f$_o$*) is always about 6 Hz

Table 1. *Summary of the results in finger tapping test in parkinsonism*

Maximal		5 Hz
Responsive	< 2 Hz	normal
	> 2.5 Hz	converging into 5 Hz
Anticipatory	> 0.5 Hz	converging into 5 Hz

Maximal: Free tapping with maximum frequency.

Responsive: When requested to tap in response to given signals of various frequency.

Anticipatory: Signal of various frequency is given for seconds and suddenly stopped, requesting the examiner to continue in the same frequency. This is more difficult for the patient, when the signal is of more than 0.5 Hz and tapping rate quickly converges into 5 Hz.

However, the neural mechanism and the metabolic background underlying such very specific pattern of rhythm formation in parkinsonism is still unknown. It must be noted that the author and his colleagues have first described the series of cases which presented solely such freezing phenomenon in gait, speech and handwriting without any sign of rigidity and tremor from the first beginning and throughout the course of the disease [8]. These cases are considered idiopathic in etiology and the above-described disturbance of rhythm formation was clearly demonstrated, thus being named by the author as "cases of pure akinesia", which was assumed to be different condition from parkinsonism.

References

[1] *Barbeau, A.:* Contributions of levodopa therapy to the neurophar-macology of akinesia. In: Parkinson's Disease, Vol. 1 (*Siegfried, J.,* ed.), pp. 151—174. Bern: Huber. 1972.

[2] *Hornykiewicz, O.:* Biochemical and pharmacological aspects of akinesia. In: Parkinson's Disease, Vol. 1 (*Siegfried, J.,* ed.), pp. 127 to 149. Bern: Huber. 1972.

[3] *Hughes, R. C., Polgar, J. G., Weightman, D., Walton, J. N.:* L-dopa in parkinsonism and the influence of previous thalamotomy. Brit. med. J. *1*, 7—13 (1974).

[4] *Imai, H., Narabayashi, H.:* Akinesia (Jap.). Advanc. neurol. Sci. *18*, 787—794 (1974).

[5] *Martin, Z. P.:* The Basal Ganglia and Posture, pp. 7—19 and pp. 52 to 54.

[6] *Nakamura, R., Nagasaki, H., Narabayashi, H.:* Arrhythmokinesia in parkinsonism. In: Advances in Parkinsonism (*Birkmayer, W., et al.,* eds.), pp. 258—268. Basle: Roche. 1976.

[7] *Nakamura, R., Nagasaki, H., Narabayashi, H.:* Disturbances of rhythm formation in patients with Parkinson's disease: Pt. 1. Charac-teristics of tapping response to the periodic signals. Percept. Motor Skills *46*, 63—75 (1978).

[8] *Narabayashi, H., Imai, H., Yokochi, M., Hirayama, K., Nakamura, R.:* Cases of pure akinesia without rigidity and tremor and with no effect by L-dopa therapy. In: Advances in Parkinsonism (*Birkmayer, W., et al.,* eds.), pp. 335—342. Basle: Roche. 1976.

[9] *Narabayashi, H., Ohye, C.:* Parkinsonian tremor and nucleus ventralis intermedius of the human thalamus. In: Progress in Clinical Neuro-physiology, Vol. 5 (*Desmedt, J. E.,* ed.), pp. 165—172. Basel: Karger. 1978.

[10] *Ohye, C., Tsukahara, N., Narabayashi, H.:* Rigidity and disturbance of reciprocal innervation. Confin. neurol. *26*, 24—40 (1965).

[11] *Wertham, F. I.:* A new sign of cerebellar disease. J. nerv. ment. Dis. *69*, 486—493 (1929).

Author's address: *H. Narabayashi*, M.D., Department of Neurology, Juntendo Medical School, 2-1-1 Hongo, Bunkyo-ku, Tokyo, Japan.

Journal of Neural Transmission, Suppl. 16, 137—141 (1980)
© by Springer-Verlag 1980

Akinetic Freezing and Trick Movements in Parkinson's Disease

G. M. Stern, C. M. Lander, and A. J. Lees

Department of Neurology, University College Hospital, London, U.K.

Summary

The clinical features of akinetic freezing occurring in a group of 85 patients with idiopathic Parkinsonism and the individual methods used to overcome immobility are described. Frequency and severity of attacks are related to duration of disease and are not amenable to currently available medications. The pathogenesis and therapeutic implications are briefly discussed.

Introduction

It has long been recognised that almost all of the signs, symptoms and disabilities of Parkinsonism may show considerable diurnal fluctuations. Of these incapacities, an abrupt inability to initiate voluntary movement particularly walking is probably the most distressing and humiliating. Patients and their families employ a variety of synonyms but commonly say that their legs are inexplicably "frozen to the spot". This state of complete immobility and helplessness may last for seconds, minutes and occasionally for hours when equally abruptly the capacity for movement may return. Akinetic freezing usually occurs independently of the oscillations or performance which are described under the rubric of "on-off" phenomena and tend to be more hazardous, often culminating in falls. Many sufferers maintain that there is a strong link with external trigger factors which may provoke as well as relieve freezing episodes, but the association is not invariable. Since the levodopa era patients have survived longer and akinetic freezing is witnessed more frequently. Attacks seem to be unrelated to the timing of individual doses of medication, but tend to occur, albeit unpredictably, when the patient is physically tired.

10*

In an attempt to overcome their enforced immobility, patients and their attendants have described many manoeuvres, stratagems or tricks and these have attracted the attentions of many clinicians. Thus in 1932, Luria described in considerable detail a patient who became completely immobile whenever he attempted to walk on an even surface, but who could easily run upstairs. He concluded from this and from other instances that it should be possible to make practical and therapeutic use of this paradox (akinesia paradoxa) which could be implemented into methods of physiotherapy and rehabilitation—"the healthy cortex enables the Parkinsonian patient to use external stimuli and to construct a compensatory activity for subcortical automatism". *Purdon Martin* (1967) summarized his extensive investigations into disordered gait, balance and posture in patients with post-encephalitic disease and drew particular attention to the potential benefit that might be gained from parallel spaced white lines and similar visual-spatial clues. More recently *Sacks* (1976) also discussed the strategems employed by post-encephalitic patients to overcome akinetic freezing. The variety and effectiveness of tricks discovered and employed by patients in attempting to overcome this disability is sparsely documented and prompted the present study.

Methods and Results

85 patients with idiopathic Parkinson's disease completed a postal questionary concerning akinetic freezing and the majority of patients were subsequently interviewed so that histories could be confirmed and amplified. All, except two patients who were recently diagnosed and untreated, had taken levodopa preparations for many months. Questions were specifically

Table 1

	Patients without "Freezing"	Patients with "Freezing"
Number	24	61
Sex	8 Female 16 Male	29 Female 32 Male
Age	Mean 65 years Range: 36—80	Mean 65.2 years Range: 45—82
Mean duration of disease	5 years Range: 1 1/2—14	12.3 years Range: 3—24
Mean duration of L-dopa treatment	2.9 years Range: 0—9	7.0 years Range: 0—9

directed to the nature, frequency and circumstances of freezing episodes and the action taken by patients to overcome immobility. 61 confirmed their vulnerability to incapacitating freezing and their salient clinical features are set out in Table 1. Clearly the longer the duration of the disease the more likely are such attacks to occur. Precipitating circumstances varied widely and seemed to include almost every possible daily activity. 60 patients stated that freezing was more likely to occur when they wished to begin walking, change direction of gait, when turning or when attempting to arise from a chair; 20 stressed the significance of people or physical obstacles in their pathway or when manoeuvring in confined spaces such as doorways and lifts; 12 emphasised the significance of surprise or sudden anxieties in provoking an attack. Other common pre-disposing factors

Table 2

	Number of patients
A. Gait modification by unaccompanied patient	
Altering distribution of body weight	4
Walking sideways "crablike"	4
Rocking movements of body	3
Stamping feet or shaking legs	2
Longer steps; walking briskly	2
Consciously lifting one limb higher	1
Sliding one foot backwards then throwing it forwards	1
B. Assisted by another person	
Rhythmical pulling or pushing	2
Passively elevating patient's knee	1
C. Verbal or auditory stimuli	
Marching to command like a soldier	13
Walking or dancing to music or metronome	5
Another person giving verbal commands	3
Sudden clapping of hands by another person	1
Swearing at himself!	1
D. Visual stimuli	
Stepping over objects, including end of walking stick, another person's foot, paving stone, carpet patterns	7
Watching other people walk	3
Pushing an object e.g. chair, block of wood, in front of foot	1
Imagining white lines to step over	1
E. Other stimuli	
Complex postural movements associated with clicking of fingers	1
Sudden jerky head movements	1

included walking on contrasting surfaces such as from tile to carpet, fatigue
or a particular physical effort such as unscrewing a tight jar. 7 mentioned
that freezing was more likely to occur on arising in the morning. Of the
61 patients afflicted with incapacitating freezing, 14 had discovered no trick
to abort or overcome their symptom. Of the remaining 47, 16 commented
on the necessity of attempting to concentrate on rhythmical walking
movements in conjunction with certain manoeuvres and 8 of these emphasized that if their concentration was interrupted their trick manoeuvre
would not be effective. Patients often resorted to more than one method;
these we set out in Table 2. However, all the patients except 8 admitted that
their tricks were not always effective in overcoming immobility nor could
attacks be prevented or the frequency reduced. The most that could be
reasonably anticipated was to shorten the duration of immobility.

Illustrative Case Histories

Case 1: An intelligent 70 year old man with a seven year history of
Parkinson's disease had taken levodopa for five years. For eighteen months
he found that his legs would unpredictably freeze at least twelve times a day.
An unexpected knock at the door would reduce him to a state of complete
immobility and he had taught himself to make no effort to move when
disturbed. He had noticed that if he was engaged in lively conversation
or intellectually distracted he was far less likely to suffer attacks.

Case 2: A 69 year old man with a ten year history of Parkinson's disease
had taken levodopa for nine years. He began to develop freezing episodes
three years ago which became so severe and frequent that he was no longer
able to live independently. It is now impossible for him to take more than
three or four steps without freezing and he is unable to climb into a lift.
He has little or no difficulty with stairs which he climbs briskly. His
attacks are unrelated to the timing of his medications and he has employed
with varying success a variety of manoeuvres. If he is alone, he deliberately
places his weight on his left leg, slowly slides his right foot backwards, then
abruptly swings it forwards in an attempt to initiate walking movement.
He estimates that this manoeuvre is successful about half of the time. He
was introduced to the technique of stepping over the end of his projected
walking stick, but this only caused him to trip and fall. However if he is
accompanied by his wife he can usually manage to successfully step over
her outstretched foot and initiate smooth walking movements.

Discussion

Elucidating the details of how long and individual has suffered
from freezing, how a particular trick had been discovered and it's
true effectiveness proved to be difficult in many patients. The re-
curring obstacle was the presence of memory impairment in many
patients with longstanding disease; this may be relevant to impaired

concentration when attempting to interrupt a freezing episode. Perhaps there are potential opportunities for the design of bio-mechanical triggering devices based on the metronome principle which might rhythmically enhance waning concentration (certain patients claimed relief by singing marches to themselves). While there are other limitations to the accuracy of information gained from question-naires in Parkinsonians, we have little doubt that the longer the duration of disease the more frequent and incapacitating are akinetic freezing episodes. In our experience, levodopa therapy with or with-out a peripheral decarboxylase inhibitor or a selective monoamine oxidase inhibitor is of little value in favourably influencing these particular disabilities.

We were disappointed with the overall effectiveness of trick movements. While benefit may be evident and at times dramatic when a trick is first demonstrated or practised, it rarely proves to be of sustained value. While a minority of enterprising patients discover a sequence of idiosyncratic manoeuvres to replace those no longer effective, for the majority of patients as their disease progresses, freezing episodes become more frequent and more difficult to overcome. The pathogenesis of akinetic freezing and the limited effectiveness of trick movements remains cryptic. Current notions, which refer mainly to altered states of sensitivity in dopaminergic receptors, intermittent and varying availability of dopamine and blockade by false neurotransmitters may prove to be too simple and facile. The influence and mechanisms of associated psychological factors also require explanation. Perhaps the fluctuating and complex influence of other neurotransmitter systems—known, putative or as yet unsuspected—may eventually provide a more comprehensible explanation, hopefully amenable to treatment. That the motor system of an immobile, incapacitated patient can be suddenly switched to useful activity provides one of the most challenging yet encouraging unresolved problems for all those engaged in the field of extrapyramidal disorders.

References

Luria, A. R.: The Nature of Human Conflicts, 1st ed., p. 153. Liverghite. 1932.

Martin, J. P.: The Basal Ganglia and Posture, 1st ed., p. 33. London: Pitman. 1967.

Sacks, O. W.: Awakenings, 2nd ed., p. 318. London: Pelican. 1976.

Authors' address: Dr. *G. M. Stern,* University College Hospital, London, WC1E 6 AU, U.K.

Journal of Neural Transmission, Suppl. 16, 143—148 (1980)

Distribution and Metabolism of the Potential Anti-Parkinson Drug Memantine in the Human

W. Wesemann, G. Sturm, and E. W. Fünfgeld

Abteilung für Neurochemie, Physiologisch-Chemisches Institut II, Philipps-Universität, Marburg/Lahn, Universitätsfrauenklinik, Philipps-Universität, Marburg/Lahn, Psychiatrisches Krankenhaus, Marburg/Lahn, Federal Republic of Germany

Summary

GC-MS of tissue extracts obtained from a parkinsonian patient who died from secondary causes during memantine (1-amino-3.5-dimethyl-adamantane) treatment showed the drug to be largely unmetabolized. In the kidney and liver a second peak corresponded to less than 1 % of the main peak. In the brain an accumulation of memantine could be shown in the temporal lobe, hypothalamus and pons. Thus treatment with 2×10 mg memantine/day reveals an accumulation of the drug in μM concentrations in the brain. This is probably high enough to explain the ameliorating effect of memantine treatment in patients suffering from Parkinson's disease.

Introduction

The adamantane derivative memantine (1-amino-3.5-dimethyl-adamantane) was shown to have beneficial influence on rigor and tremor of parkinsonian patients (*Fünfgeld*, 1976; *Fischer et al.*, 1977) and on rigor and spasticity of different origin (*Fünfgeld*, 1975). The effect of memantine may be explained by dopamine receptor stimulation (*Svensson*, 1973; *Maj et al.*, 1974) and by a decrease in the conduction of nerve membranes for Na^+, K^+ and Cl^- (*Grossmann* and *Jurna*, 1977). Moreover it could be demonstrated by *in vitro* experiments that memantine induces the release of 5-HT and DA from isolated nerve endings. Since subthreshold concentrations of this drug (5—50 μM), which are too low to liberate the transmitter, increase the electrical stimulated release, memantine may act in parkinsonian patient by enriching the transmitter content in the synaptic cleft (*Wesemann et al., 1979*).

The present studies were performed in order to elucidate if after treatment of parkinsonian patients with memantine the enrichment of the drug in the brain is high enough to induce increased transmitter release. Thus the distribution of memantine was studied in different brain areas and 6 other organs of a memantine treated parkinsonian patient who died after a sudden heart failure. In addition, the metabolism of the drug was investigated in order to exclude the possibility that metabolites are responsible for the favourable effects observed after memantine treatment.

Materials and Methods

1. Drug

MemantineINN (1-amino-3.5-dimethyladamantane) was kindly provided by Merz & Co., Frankfurt/Main, Federal Republic of Germany.

2. Case History and Autopsy

A 77-year woman with arteriosclerotic Parkinson syndrome was hospitalized since 1974. Signs of cerebral arteriosclerosis, hypertonia, and a marked akinesia were prominent during the first 2 years. Rigor developed in the third year, the difficulty in swallowing augmented. Therapy with cardiacs, xantinolnicotinat, opipramol and—later—with baclofen and pyridostigminbromid showed no influences at all. Baclofen treatment was stopped 1977. A few days after beginning of memantine treatment the rigor was markedly diminished. Moreover the patient's apathy and lack of interests were much more reduced than during the previous therapeutical trials. This was also obvious during the physiotherapist's exercises. During the further treatment with memantine, opipramol and pyridostigminbromid therapy were arrested without any negative influences. A cardiac infarct and edema of the lungs were the possible causes of death. The patient was on memantine treatment for 59 days before death (10 mg daily for 6 days, followed by 2×10 mg daily for 53 days). The last 10 mg memantine were administered one hour before death. About 3 hours elapsed between death and refrigeration (4 °C). Autopsy was performed 26 hours after death. Brain was immediately dissected after removal from the skull. Brain tissue and the other organs were deep frozen at —70 °C until analysis (within 1 month).

3. Assay of Memantine

Tissue was homogenized in 10 vol. of 0.1 N HCl using a potter with glass pistil. Kidney, spleen, and heart were minced with a Waring blender prior to homogenization. The extraction of memantine and possible metabolites was performed as described earlier (*Wesemann et al.*, 1977). Briefly this includes titration of the samples with 2 N NaOH to pH 11—12, extraction with n-heptane and removal of water by freezing (—20 °C).

Gas-liquid-chromatography was performed with a Hewlett-Packard model 5830 A gaschromatograph fitted with an FID. Separation was achieved using a 3 m glass column, 2 mm i.d., packed with 2 % Dexsil 300 on Gaschrom P 80—100 mesh. The flow rate of the N_2 carrier gas was 35 ml/min, injection temperature 210 °C, FID 230 °C, oven temperature 100 °C with temperature programme 6 °C/min to 190 °C.

Mass spectra were obtained with identical GC conditions with the exception that shorter columns, 1.5 m, i.d. 2 mm, were used which were packed either with 2 % Dexsil 300 or 3 % SE 30 on Gaschrom P. The carrier gas was helium, 30 ml/min. A Dupont 21-492 B mass spectrometer with Varian GC 1400 and one step jet separator as well as a Varian MAT 711 with Varian GC 2700 and two step Watson Beamann separator were used, separator temperature 250 °C, ion source ca. 250 °C.

External standards were applied for quantitative analysis of memantine levels in the tissue extracts. The calibration curve was linear from 15 to 300 pg memantine/μl.

Results and Discussion

The gaschromatograms of the tissue extracts showed mainly one intense peak. However, in the extracts of kidney and liver, a second, very small peak was observed. The area of this peak corresponded to less than 1 % of the main peak.

The main peak could be identified by GC/MS as unmetabolized memantine. Besides the molecular ion at m/e 179 the fragment ion at m/e 164 was found which could be explained by elimination of one methyl group. The most intensive mass peaks were found at m/e 108 ($C_7H_{10}N$) and at m/e 122 ($C_8H_{12}N$), which correspond to the loss of C_5H_{11} and C_4H_9, respectively.

The analysis of the different tissues indicate that, as compared with other organs, rather high memantine concentrations are accumulated in the brain, especially in temporal lobe, hypothalamus, and pons (Table 1).

Assuming that memantine is equally distributed between the different cell compartments and that in brain 1 g wet weight corresponds to 1 ml, a very rough calculation of the molar memantine concentrations can be performed. The values obtained by this calculation (Table 1, third column) ranging from 0.5 μM memantine for the central motoric region to 1.8 μM memantine for the temporal lobe are certainly lower than the actual concentrations in the biophase since adamantanes are known to be incorporated into membranes as was shown for, *e.g.*, by spin label experiments with liposomes (*Eletr*

Table 1. *Distribution of 1-amino-3.5-dimethyladamantane (memantine) in human brain and other tissues*

Tissue	Concentration of memantine	
	μg/g wet weight	μM*
Temporal lobe	0.39	1.80
Hypothalamus	0.31	1.43
Pons	0.31	1.41
Frontal lobe	0.28	1.29
Caput N.C. + putamen	0.24	1.13
Thalamus	0.22	1.04
Cerebellum	0.22	1.03
Premotoric region	0.22	1.03
Medulla	0.21	0.96
Postcentral-parietal + occipital region	0.15	0.71
Central motoric region	0.11	0.49
Kidney	0.18	0.83
Lung	0.17	0.80
Spleen	0.10	0.48
Heart	0.08	0.37
Blood	0.07	0.32
Liver	0.01	0.06

* The molar concentrations are calculated on the basis that memantine is equally distributed between all cell compartments of each tissue and that 1 g tissue wet weight corresponds to 1 ml.

77 year old woman, treated with 10 mg memantine[INN]/day for 6 days, followed by 2×10 mg memantine for 53 days; last dose given 1 hour before death.

The values given are the mean of two extractions, each examined three times; SD ± 5.3 %.

et al., 1964; *Cupp et al.*, 1975). On the basis that memantine is evenly distributed between all kinds of lipids in white and grey matter (ca. 15 % of brain fresh weight are lipids) the molar concentrations given in Table 1 are to be raised by factor 6—7. Since studies on the subcellular distribution of memantine in brain have not yet been published the calculated molar concentrations cannot be used as absolute values. They indicate however, that under chronic treatment with 2×10 mg memantine/day the drug is accumulated in μM concentrations. According to the above mentioned *in vitro* experiments these concentrations are high enough to enhance transmitter release into the synaptic cleft on presynaptic stimulation. This finding might explain the ameliorating effect of memantine treatment in patients suffering from M. Parkinson.

Similarly, the relatively high memantine concentrations found in kidney and lung may reflect the importance of these two organs in memantine excretion. This view is supported by previous findings of *Bleidner et al.* (1965) on the essential role of kidney and lung for the excretion of 1-aminoadamantane, the unmethylated parent compound of memantine. In addition, the importance of the kidney for excretion of memantine and its metabolites was already demonstrated (*Wesemann et al.*, 1977). Though surprisingly low concentrations of memantine were found in liver, in addition to the main memantine peak a second peak was found in gaschromatograms of liver extracts. The retention time of this small peak was identical with that of the one found in gaschromatograms of the kidney. This peak was also observed in gaschromatograms of urine extracts from a patient treated with 1×10 mg memantine per day and from a volunteer receiving one single 10 mg dose of this drug. By means of mass fragmentography the small peak could be identified as 1-amino-3-hydroxymethyl-5-methyl-adamantane (M^+: m/e 195, 164, 138, 124, 108). Neither this metabolite nor other hydroxylderivatives of memantine, which could be demonstrated in the urine of rats under treatment, were detectable in the analysed brain regions (*Wesemann et al.*, 1977). The results suggest that hydroxylated metabolites which are likely to be synthesized in liver, do not permeate the blood-brain barrier but are excreted by the kidney in the urine. Since the presence as well as the metabolization and distribution of the metabolites within the body depend on the administered dose, future studies using rats should elucidate the influence of the applied dose on these parameters.— However, in the case reported here, it is very unlikely that metabolites are responsible for the observed beneficial effect of memantine treatment since no hydroxylderivatives could be detected in the brain.

Acknowledgements

The authors would like to thank Miss V. Süwer for excellent technical assistance. They are also grateful to Drs. Peteri and Scherm of Merz & Co., Frankfurt/Main, for the generous supply of memantine.—This work was supported by the Deutsche Forschungsgemeinschaft.

References

Bleidner, W. E., Harmon, J. B., Hewes, W. E., Lynes, T. E., Hermann, E. C.: Absorption, distribution and excretion of amantadine hydrochloride. J. Pharmacol. Exp. Therap. *150*, 484—490 (1965).

Cupp, J., Klymkowski, M., Sands, J., Keith, A., Snipes, W.: Effect of lipid alkyl chain perturbations on the assembly of bacteriophage PM 2. Biochim. Biophys. Acta 389, 345—357 (1975).

Eletr, S., Williams, M. A., Watkins, T., Keith, A. D.: Perturbations of the dynamics of lipid alkyl chains in membrane systems: Effect on the activity of membrane-bound enzymes. Biochim. Biophys. Acta 339, 190—201 (1974).

Fischer, P.-A., Jacobi, P., Schneider, E., Schönberger, B.: Die Wirkung intravenöser Gaben von Memantin bei Parkinson-Kranken. Arzneim.-Forsch. (Drug Res.) 27, 1487—1489 (1977).

Fünfgeld, E. W.: 33 Monate Therapie mit Dimethylaminoadamantan. Unpublished paper (1975).

Fünfgeld, E. W.: Konservative Behandlung des Parkinsonismus. Vortrag und Film. Medizin. Gesellschaft Freiburg/Breisgau, February 3, 1976.

Grossmann, W., Jurna, I.: Die Wirkung von Memantin auf die Membranen sensibler Nervenfaserbündel. Arzneim.-Forsch. (Drug Res.) 27, 1483 to 1487 (1977).

Maj, J., Marchaj, J., Mogilnicka, E.: The effect of dimethyladamantane on the brain 5-hydroxytryptamine and 5-hydroxyindoleacetic acid levels. Second Congr. Hung. Pharmacol. Soc. Budapest, 1974. Cited from: Maj, J.: Dopaminergic drugs and serotonin neurons. In: Current Developments in Psychopharmacology (Essman, W. B., Valzelli, L., eds.), Vol. 3, pp. 55—83. New York-Toronto-London-Sydney: Spectrum. 1976.

Svensson, T. H.: Dopamine release and direct dopamine receptor activation in the central nervous system by D 145, an amantadine derivative. Eur. J. Pharmacol. 23, 232—238 (1973).

Wesemann, W., Schollmeyer, J. D., Sturm, G.: Gaschromatographische und massenspektrometrische Untersuchungen über harnpflichtige Metaboliten von Adamantanaminen. Arzneim.-Forsch. (Drug Res.) 27, 1471—1476 (1977).

Wesemann, W., Dette-Wildenhahn, G., Fellehner, H.: In vitro studies on the possible effects of 1-aminoadamantanes on the serotonergic system in M. Parkinson. J. Neural Transm. 44, 263—285 (1979).

Authors' address: Prof. Dr. W. Wesemann, Abteilung für Neurochemie, Physiologisch-Chemisches Institut II, Philipps-Universität, D-3550 Marburg/Lahn, Federal Republic of Germany.

Journal of Neural Transmission, Suppl. 16, 149—156 (1980)

Long-Term Responses of Parkinson's Disease to Levodopa Therapy

U. K. Rinne, V. Sonninen, T. Siirtola, and R. Marttila

Department of Neurology, University of Turku, Turku, Finland

Summary

The long-term responses of Parkinson's disease to levodopa therapy were studied in the patient material followed-up for 9 years. Levodopa treatment alleviated the parkinsonian symptoms to a considerable degree and substantially improved the quality of life of the parkinsonian patients. However, after treatment for 2 to 3 years, a progressive deterioration of parkinsonian symptoms was observed accompanied by an increase in the incidence of dyskinesias, on-off phenomena, postural instability and dementia. An analysis of the mortality rates in the follow-up material of 349 patients showed that initially levodopa treatment decreased the excess mortality due to Parkinson's disease. The ratios of observed to expected deaths ranged from 1.10 to 1.67. However, during the ninth year of treatment the ratio increased to 1.95 almost reaching the values obtained in the first years of levodopa treatment. Thus it appears that levodopa has only a limited period of usefulness in the treatment of Parkinson's disease. Although levodopa very significantly improves parkinsonian symptoms, it does not arrest the pathological progress and modify the natural course of the disease.

Levodopa treatment with or without a decarboxylase inhibitor alleviates the symptoms of Parkinson's disease to a considerable degree and substantially improves the quality of life of parkinsonian patients (*Barbeau*, 1969; *Birkmayer*, 1969; *Cotzias et al.*, 1969; *Yahr et al.*, 1969; *Rinne et al.*, 1970). However, in spite of a good initial response, a progressive deterioration of parkinsonian symptoms has been observed after treatment with levodopa for several years, associated at the same time with an increase in the incidence of long-term side effects of levodopa treatment (see: *Rinne*, 1978).

In this paper we would like to describe our results on the responses of parkinsonian patients to long-term levodopa therapy.

Results

Long-Term Therapeutic Efficacy

The responses of parkinsonian clinical features to long-term combined treatment of up to 9 years with levodopa and a decarboxylase inhibitor, benserazide, are shown in Table 1. There is a significant improvement in the clinical condition of the patients during the first 6 months of the treatment. However, in spite of a good initial response for 2 to 3 years, with the passage of time the patients on long-term levodopa treatment begin to lose the initial benefit. Indeed, the parkinsonian disability seems to return to the pretreatment level after 7 years' treatment. The deterioration of tremor was not as permanent as that of other symptoms.

As can be seen from Table 2, the long-term response to levodopa seems to be variable in different subgroups of the patients. Sixteen per cent of our parkinsonian patients treated with levodopa and benserazide maintained their initial benefit for years and showed only minimal worsening, whereas 20 per cent of the patients showed marked deterioration already after one year's treatment and within 4 years they had lost all the initial benefit. Accordingly, the first subgroup of patients could be called the benign type and the second one the malignant type of idiopathic Parkinson's disease. The remaining 64 per cent of the patients had moderate deterioration during long-term levodopa treatment but after 9 years of treatment are still better than they were before the onset of therapy.

Table 3 shows that there are some significant differences between these subgroups of long-term levodopa response. Patients with the malignant type of the disease had a significantly shorter duration of the disease and less severe pretreatment severity of the disease at entry than others.

An analysis of factors governing a patient's response to chronic levodopa treatment showed that initially there was a negative correlation between the pretreatment severity of the disease and the improvement of the patients during the first 3 years of treatment with levodopa. However, during the subsequent deterioration of the parkinsonian disability on chronic levodopa treatment, this relationship seems to become even inverse (Table 4).

Together with a deteriorating levodopa response the most distressing problem during chronic levodopa treatment seems to be the daily

Table 1. *Improvement (%) of parkinsonian patients during long-term treatment with levodopa and benserazide. Mean ± S.E.M.*

Variable	Duration of treatment (years)								
	1	2	3	4	5	6	7	8	9
Total disability	47±3 (65)	46±3 (76)	40±4 (51)	32±4 (50)	24±4 (60)	16±4 (57)	10±4 (46)	2± 5 (32)	-10± 8 (13)
Tremor	54±4 (65)	56±4 (75)	51±5 (50)	45±7 (49)	37±7 (61)	34±7 (57)	34±7 (47)	27±11 (32)	30±13 (13)
Rigidity	44±3 (65)	35±4 (76)	27±6 (50)	22±6 (50)	9±5 (61)	3±6 (57)	-10±7 (47)	-24± 8 (32)	-34±14 (13)
Hypokinesia	51±3 (65)	48±4 (75)	44±5 (51)	31±5 (50)	26±5 (61)	20±4 (57)	6±7 (47)	-2± 8 (32)	-12± 8 (13)

Table 2. *Improvement (%) of parkinsonian patients during long-term treatment with levodopa and benserazide. Responses of different subgroups of the patients. Mean ± S.E.M.*

Subgroup of response	Duration of treatment (years)								
	1	2	3	4	5	6	7	8	9
Marked improvement, minimal worsening	58±7 (14)	61±7 (14)	62±6 (14)	57±6 (14)	53±5 (14)	46±6 (14)	37±6 (10)	34±11 (5)	14± 0 (1)
Moderate improvement and worsening	48±3 (45)	46±3 (53)	41±4 (45)	39±3 (36)	28±3 (30)	17±3 (30)	12±4 (26)	5± 4 (19)	3± 5 (8)
Moderate improvement and marked worsening	38±5 (11)	33±7 (14)	19±7 (14)	3±7 (13)	-9±6 (16)	-20±4 (13)	-27±9 (10)	-26± 7 (8)	-42±15 (4)

Table 3. *Clinical variables of subgroups of response to long-term treatment with levodopa and benserazide of 87 parkinsonian patients followed up for up to 9 years*

Subgroup of response	Number of patients (%)	Age at entry (years)	Duration of disease at entry (years)	Pretreatment severity							Frequency	
				Total score	Disability stage						AIM (%)	"On-off" (%)
					I (%)	II	III	IV	V			
Marked improvement, minimal worsening	16	57±2.9	7.6±1.1	52±4	—	14	57	29	—		93	50
Moderate improvement and worsening	64	63±1.1	6.7±0.9	52±2	4	18	44	30	4		75	43
Moderate improvement, marked worsening	20	58±1.5	4.0±0.7	41±2	6	35	47	12	—		65	65
P 1—2		<0.05		<0.05	<0.05						n.s.	n.s.
P 1—3			<0.05	<0.001	<0.01						n.s.	n.s.
P 2—3		<0.05	<0.05								n.s.	n.s.

Table 4. *Improvement (%) of parkinsonian patients during long-term treatment with levodopa and benserazide. Relationship between pretreatment stage of the disease and improvement. Mean ± S.E.M.*

Stage of the disease*	Duration of treatment (years)								
	1	2	3	4	5	6	7	8	9
I and II	57±5 (14)	55±6 (20)	50±8 (18)	34±7 (18)	23±8 (18)	10±8 (17)	8±9 (15)	-1±10 (11)	-14±23 (4)
III	51±3 (34)	45±4 (37)	38±5 (35)	34±6 (30)	23±6 (32)	18±5 (30)	7±6 (24)	3±6 (16)	-12±8 (7)
IV and V	35±4 (21)	39±5 (23)	35±6 (19)	36±5 (14)	27±6 (11)	20±7 (10)	22±7 (8)	3±13 (5)	6±5 (2)

* According to *Hoehn* and *Yahr* (1967).

fluctuations in performance. In our follow-up material these on-off phenomena were increasingly more frequent within the time of treatment and involved about half of the patients after 7—9 years of treatment with levodopa and benserazide. From various patterns contributing to on-off disturbances during long-term treatment with levodopa, the end-of-dose disturbances (60 %) and freezing episodes (70 %) were the most frequent ones. Other difficulties during long-term levodopa treatment included dyskinesias, postural instability and mental changes, especially loss of memory together with a declining intellectual capacity.

Mortality

To clarify whether long-term levodopa treatment increases the life span of parkinsonian patients by decreasing the excess mortality due to the disease, the mortality of parkinsonian patients under chronic levodopa therapy was investigated. During the follow-up period from 1969 to 1978, 109 patients (44 women and 65 men) died out of the 349 parkinsonian patients followed. The calculated expected mortality for the whole period was 30.79 for women and 37.60 for men, resulting in a ratio of observed to expected deaths of 1.43 for women and 1.73 for men, and 1.59 for both sexes combined (Table 5).

When the ratios of observed to expected deaths were calculated for different years, it was found that during the first 4 years the number of observed deaths was more than twice the expected deaths, but during subsequent years the excess mortality clearly decreased, the ratios ranging from 1.10 to 1.67. However, during 1978 the mortality of the patients again increased, reaching almost the levels obtained in the first years of levodopa treatment (Table 5).

Conclusions

The long-term follow-up of parkinsonian patients showed that levodopa treatment significantly improves the quality of life of parkinsonian patients for several years. However, after a successful period of maintenance treatment of varying length, various difficulties become evident during chronic levodopa therapy, *e.g.* loss of benefit, dyskinesias, on-off phenomena, postural instability and declining intellectual capacity.

Although the initial therapeutic response to levodopa significantly depends on the pretreatment severity of the disease, this seems not to be the case for the decrease of benefit derived from levodopa during

Table 5. *Mortality of patients with Parkinson's disease treated with levodopa*

Year	Females			Males			Total		
	Observed	Expected	Ratio	Observed	Expected	Ratio	Observed	Expected	Ratio
1969—1971	7	2.91	2.41	10	5.10	1.96	17	8.01	2.12
1972	4	2.49	1.61	11	3.29	3.34	15	5.78	2.60
1973	4	2.96	1.35	4	3.76	1.06	8	6.72	1.19
1974	5	3.51	1.42	5	4.56	1.10	10	8.07	1.24
1975	3	4.03	0.74	8	5.33	1.50	11	9.36	1.18
1976	8	4.74	1.69	9	5.42	1.67	17	10.16	1.67
1977	3	4.85	0.62	8	5.18	1.54	11	10.03	1.10
1978	10	5.30	1.89	10	4.96	2.02	20	10.26	1.95
Total	44	30.79	1.43	65	37.60	1.73	109	68.39	1.59

long-term treatment. Furthermore, our follow-up data of different subgroups of response to chronic levodopa therapy suggest that there are different types of idiopathic Parkinson's disease, possibly associated with the different rates of progression of nigral cell loss, although differences in response cannot completely account for it.

An analysis of the mortality rates in the present follow-up material indicated that levodopa treatment decreases the excess mortality accompanying the natural course of Parkinson's disease. Before the introduction of levodopa treatment this excess mortality was found to be three times that expected in the general population of the same age and sex (*Hoehn* and *Yahr*, 1967). Attempts to analyse retrospectively the excess mortality have yielded similar figures (*Diamond* and *Markham*, 1976; *Marttila* and *Rinne*, 1979). On the other hand, our present mortality data show that during the first 4 years of levodopa treatment, the excess mortality was only slightly reduced. This was most probably due to the deaths of the patients, in whom the treatment was initiated at an advanced stage of the disease. During the following years, when most patients were on the maintenance phase and obtained best benefit from levodopa therapy, the mortality was reduced almost to the levels expected in the general population. It seems, however, that the reduction of the excess mortality may be temporary, since in this patient population we observed a striking increase of mortality after 5 years of low mortality. If not a fortuitous phenomenon, this may reflect the concurrently increasing incidence of long-term levodopa treatment difficulties, *e.g.* loss of benefit, on-off phenomena, postural instability, and dementia.

Thus it appears that levodopa has only a limited period of usefulness. It merely improves parkinsonian symptoms but does not modify the natural course of the disease. These aspects seriously warrant the exploration of new paths in the treatment of Parkinson's disease, especially its diverse symptoms developing during the later stages of the disease.

References

Barbeau, A.: L-Dopa therapy in Parkinson's disease. A critical review of nine years experience. Canad. med. Ass. J. *101*, 791—800 (1969).

Birkmayer, W.: Experimentelle Ergebnisse über die Kombinationsbehandlung des Parkinson-Syndroms mit L-Dopa und einem Decarboxylasehemmer (Ro 4-4602). Wien. klin. Wschr. *81*, 677—679 (1969).

Cotzias, G. C., Papavasiliou, P. S., Gellene, R.: Modification of Parkinsonism—chronic treatment with L-Dopa. N. Engl. J. Med. *280*, 337 to 345 (1969).

Diamond, S. G., Markham, Ch. H.: Present mortality in Parkinson's disease: the ratio of observed to expected deaths with a method to calculate expected deaths. J. Neural Transm. *38,* 259—269 (1976).

Hoehn, M. M., Yahr, M. D.: Parkinsonism: onset, progression and mortality. Neurology (Minneap.) *17,* 427—442 (1967).

Marttila, R. J., Rinne, U. K.: Changing epidemiology of Parkinson's disease: Predicted effects of levodopa treatment. Acta neurol. Scand. *59,* 80—87 (1979).

Rinne, U. K., Sonninen, V., Siirtola, T.: L-Dopa treatment in Parkinson's disease. Eur. Neurol. *4,* 348—369 (1970).

Rinne, U. K.: Recent advances in research on Parkinsonism. Acta neurol. Scand. *57,* 77—113 (1978).

Yahr, M. D., Duvoisin, R. C., Shear, M. J.: Treatment of parkinsonism with levodopa. Arch. Neurol. (Chic.) *21,* 343—354 (1969).

Authors' address: Prof. *U. K. Rinne,* M.D., Department of Neurology, University of Turku, SF-20520 Turku 52, Finland.

Journal of Neural Transmission, Suppl. 16, 157—161 (1980)
© by Springer-Verlag 1980

Monoamine Oxidase Inhibitors as Anti-Depressant Drugs and as Adjunct to L-Dopa Therapy of Parkinson's Disease

M. B. H. Youdim

Technion—Israel Institute of Technology, Department of Pharmacology, Faculty of Medicine, Haifa, Israel

Summary

Monoamine oxidase inhibitors have been used in psychiatric disorders for many years. However, due to the toxic side effects of the drugs they are often replaced by the tri- and tetracyclic antidepressants.

Selective monoamine oxidase inhibitors like deprenyl, however, have been tried with success as adjuvant therapy in Parkinson's disease and depression because of their ability to inhibit dopamine oxidation. Perhaps their greatest advantage is their lack of pressor response.

The advent of the tranquilizing drugs and monoamine oxidase (MAO) inhibitors brought about a definite change in the philosophy of the treatment of mental disease. At least two benefits accrued from this change in our thinking:

(1) it pointed a way towards the eventual physiological treatment of mental disease and (2) it raised the possibility that certain therapeutic concepts and techniques which had dealt successfully with disease, other than mental, could be extended and applied in the treatment of psychiatric and neurological disorders.

The concepts to which we refer concern themselves primarily with the roles of such neurotransmitters of normal or abnormal physiological functions as noradrenaline (NA), adrenaline, serotonin (5-hydroxytryptamine, 5-HT) and dopamine (DA) as well as with the variety of approaches to potentiating and inhibiting their pharmacological effects. The function of the above monoamine neurotransmitters in animal behaviour, as well as in psychiatric and certain neurological disorders, has been investigated and established. Support for a link between monoamine and neurotransmitters and mental disease is provided by the beneficial effects often achieved with drugs which interfere with metabolism and function of the above monoamines in the brain.

Alteration in brain monoamine neurotransmitters' metabolism and function can be induced by drugs during their synthesis as well as during their degradation. This paper is primarily concerned with the functional role of brain monoamine oxidase (EC 1.4.3.4.), the enzyme which is responsible for the oxidative deamination of NA, adrenaline, 5-HT and DA, in Parkinson's disease and depression.

We will consider the events that occur when drugs are used that inhibit MAO and thereby increase the concentrations of neurotransmitters 5-HT and DA in the brain of animals and human subjects. The biochemists may wonder why one wishes to increase the amount of 5-HT and DA. Investigators have (a) produced considerable evidence to suggest that depressive illness may arise from abnormalities in, and probably a deficiency of, the 5-HT content of the brain and (b) established that Parkinson's disease is a deficiency of DA in neostriatum because of lesions of DA cell bodies which arise in the substantia nigra and terminate in the caudate nucleus. Thus, perhaps a rational way to attempt treatment of these disorders would be to increase the 5-HT or DA content of the brain in order to make up the deficiency. There are several different ways in which this might be done. One would be to increase the production of these amines by giving their precursors, L-3,4-dihydroxyphenylalanine (L-Dopa) and 5-hydroxytryptophan which can cross the blood brain barrier and are subsequently decarboxylated. Another way would be to inhibit the destruction of the amines by giving MAO inhibitors. The third possibility, which constitutes the subject of the present paper, is a combination of these two (*Green et al.,* 1975, 1977; *Youdim et al.,* 1976).

The unexpected mood elevating effects of iproniazid in patients with tuberculosis and the discovery in 1952 by Zeller and his co-workers that iproniazid, which was originally used for the treatment of tuberculosis was a potent inhibitor of MAO, led to the therapeutic application of this drug in the treatment of depression. The development of other hydrazine and non-hydrazine MAO inhibitors, which could be utilized for the same purpose, was a natural consequence of these findings. However, some patients treated with MAO inhibitors developed hypertensive crises ("cheese effects") sometimes with fatal consequences. It was soon discovered that ingestion of food, including cheese, containing vasoactive substances such as tyramine and L-Dopa provoked the marked rise in blood pressure due to release of noradrenaline. What has become known as the "cheese effect" has serious-

ly limited the use of MAO inhibitors as anti-depressants or agents for
the therapeutic potentiation of L-Dopa in Parkinson's disease. However, the discovery of multiple forms of brain MAO (*Youdim et al.,*
1969, 1972; *Collins et al.,* 1970) and the advent of new MAO inhibitors possibly without the "cheese effect", which can selectively in-
activate different forms of the enzyme in the peripheral tissues as well
as in the brain have improved the prospects for successful use of these
drugs.

In 1971 *Youdim et al.* (1971) suggested the synthesis of selective
monoamine oxidase inhibitors without the "cheese effect" which can
inhibit a particular form of the enzyme. The multiple forms of MAO
have been differentiated into type A and type B but by no means is
this a universal classification because there are many examples of
exception to this rule. Of importance to the clinical use of MAO
inhibitors in man is the property of MAO activity in the brain. It is
apparent that the human brain MAO is predominantly "type B" and
the selective inhibitor of this form is the inhibitor, deprenyl (*Riederer
et al.,* 1978). Deprenyl is unique among all other inhibitors synthesized in that it does not potentiate the pressor property of tyramine
in isolated pharmacological preparations or *in vivo* (*Finberg et al.,*
1980). In fact deprenyl antagonizes the pressor property of tyramine.
These two properties of deprenyl led us to introduce this drug initially
in the treatment of Parkinson's as adjunct to L-Dopa (*Birkmayer et
al.,* 1975) and more recently in the treatment of depressive illness in
combination with 5-hydroxytryptophan (*Mendlewicz* and *Youdim,*
1978). Long term treatment of Parkinson's patient with L-Dopa
results in diminished response to L-Dopa and increased incidents of
"on-off" phenomenon. The limitations in the use of L-Dopa has led
investigators to look for other drugs. Though far from resolving all
of the therapeutic difficulties encountered with prolonged use of
L-Dopa, deprenyl is most promising among all other drugs and
appears to be a very valuable adjunctive agent for long term treatment of Parkinson's disease specially those who develop the "on-
off" phenomenon (*Birkmayer et al.,* 1977; *Lees et al.,* 1977). These
results have been confirmed by many other investigators (*Birkmayer
et al.,* 1979). In the same manner we have used deprenyl to potentiate
the anti-depressant action of 5-hydroxytryptophan (5-HTP) in the
treatment of depressive illness. The results have been very encouraging and show that deprenyl plus 5-HTP is superior to treatment
with tricyclic anti-depressant (*Mendlewicz* and *Youdim,* 1978; *Youdim* and *Mendlewicz,* 1980). The mode of action of deprenyl is best
explained by its inhibition of MAO thus making more dopamine or
serotonin available at post-synaptic receptor sites and increasing their

functional activity (*Green* and *Youdim*, 1975; *Youdim et al.*, 1976). It should be stressed that we have treated over 800 Parkinsonian and about 60 depressive patients with deprenyl. In no instance did we observe a hypertensive crisis. Recently *Elsworth et al.* (1978) have challenged patients on deprenyl with up to 400 mg of oral tyramine without observing a hypertensive crisis.

The studies with deprenyl has led us to synthesize and investigate the parmacological properties of other selective inhibitors of MAO, which would be of "type B" and would not have tyramine pressor inducing property. Of the drugs investigated and developed, one drug (AGN 1135) which has similar structure and property to deprenyl seems to be most promising among all other inhibitors (*Finberg et al.*, 1980; *Youdim*, 1980) for use as an anti-depressant or as adjunct to L-Dopa therapy of Parkinson's disease.

References

Birkmayer, W., Riederer, P., Ambrozi, L., Youdim, M. B. H.: Implications of combined treatment with Madopar and L-deprenyl in Parkinson's disease. A long term study. Lancet *1*, 439—443 (1977).

Birkmayer, W., Riederer, P., Youdim, M. B. H.: Deprenyl and Parkinson's disease. In: Clinical Neuropharmacology (*Klawans, H.*, ed.). New York: Raven Press. In press.

Birkmayer, W., Riederer, P., Youdim, M. B. H., Linauer, W.: The potentiation of the anti-akinetic effects after L-Dopa treatment by an inhibitor of MAO-B, deprenil. J. Neural Transm. *36*, 303—326 (1975).

Collins, G. G. S., Sandler, M., Williams, E. D., Youdim, M. B. H.: Multiple forms of human brain mitochondriol monoamine oxidase. Nature *225*, 817—820 (1970).

Elsworth, J. D., Glover, V., Reynolds, G. P., Sandler, M., Lees, A. J., Phuapradit, P., Shaw, K. M., Stern, G. M., Kumar, P.: Deprenyl administration in man. A selective monoamine oxidase inhibitor without the "cheese effect". Psychopharmacologia *57*, 33—38 (1978).

Finberg, J., Sabbagh, A., Youdim, M. B. H.: Pharmacology of selective acetylenic suicide inhibitors of monoamine oxidase. In: Enzymes and Neurotransmitters in Mental Disease (*Usdin, E., Sourkes, T. L., Youdim, M. B. H.*, eds.). London: J. Wiley. In press (1980).

Green, A. R., Mitchell, B., Tordoff, A., Youdim, M. B. H.: Evidence for dopamine deamination by both type A and type B monoamine oxidase in rat brain *in vivo* and for the degree of inhibition of enzyme necessary for increased functional activity of dopamine and 5-hydroxytryptamine. Brit. J. Pharmacol. *60*, 343—349 (1977).

Green, A. R., Youdim, M. B. H.: Effects of monoamine oxidase inhibition by clorgyline, deprenyl or tranylcypromine on 5-hydroxytryptamine concentration in rat brain and hyperactivity following tryptophan administration. Brit. J. Pharmacol. *55*, 415—422 (1975).

Lees, A. J., Shaw, K. M., Kohout, L. J., Stern, G. M., Elsworth, J. D., Sandler, M., Youdim, M. B. H.: Deprenyl in Parkinson's disease. Lancet 2, 791—796 (1977).

Mendlewicz, J., Youdim, M. B. H.: Anti-depressant potentiation of 5-hydroxytryptophan by L-deprenyl, an MAO "type B" inhibitor. J. Neural Transm. *43*, 279—286 (1978).

Riederer, P., Youdim, M. B. H., Rausch, W. D., Birkmayer, W., Jellinger, K., Seemann, D.: On the mode of action of L-deprenyl in the human central nervous system. J. Neural Transm. *43*, 217—226 (1978).

Youdim, M. B. H.: The use of selective monoamine oxidase "type B" inhibitors in the treatment of Parkinson's disease. In: Enzymes and Neurotransmitters in Mental Disease (*Usdin, E., Sourkes, T. L., Youdim, M. B. H.,* eds.). London: J. Wiley. In press (1980).

Youdim, M. B. H., Collins, G. G. S., Sandler, M.: Multiple forms of rat brain monoamine oxidase. Nature *223*, 626—628 (1969).

Youdim, M. B. H., Collins, G. G., Sandler, M.: Monoamine oxidase: Multiple forms and selective inhibition. Biochem. J. *121*, 34—36 (1971).

Youdim, M. B. H., Collins, G. G. S., Sandler, M., Bevan Jones, A. B., Pare, C. M. B., Nicholson, W. J.: Human brain monoamine oxidase multiple forms and selective inhibitors. Nature *236*, 225—228 (1972).

Youdim, M. B. H., Green, A. R., Grahame-Smith, D. G.: The role of 5-hydroxytryptamine, dopamine and MAO in the production of hyperactivity syndrome. In: Advances in Parkinsonism (*Birkmayer, W., Hornykiewicz, O.,* eds.), pp. 155—162. Basle: Editiones Roche. 1976.

Youdim, M. B. H., Mendlewicz, J.: Monoamine oxidase inhibition without the "cheese effect": Clinical and pharmacological relevance in the treatment of depression. In: Enzymes and Neurotransmitters in Mental Disease (*Usdin, E., Sourkes, T. L., Youdim, M. B. H.,* eds.). London: J. Wiley. In press (1980).

Author's address: Prof. Dr. *M. B. H. Youdim,* Department of Pharmacology, Technion—Israel Institute of Technology, Faculty of Medicine, Haifa, Israel.

Journal of Neural Transmission, Suppl. 16, 163—172 (1980)
© by Springer-Verlag 1980

Dopamine Oxidation and Its Inhibition
by (—)-Deprenyl in Man

Vivette Glover, J. D. Elsworth, and M. Sandler

Bernhard Baron Memorial Research Laboratories and Institute of Obstetrics and Gynaecology, Queen Charlotte's Maternity Hospital, London, U.K.

With 1 Figure

Summary

Dopamine is predominantly oxidized by a (—)-deprenyl sensitive form of MAO in the human striatum, and (—)-deprenyl, acting at some suitably low selective inhibitory concentration may, therefore, be of benefit in Parkinson's disease. 10^{-6} M was the most effective (—)-deprenyl concentration *in vitro* for discriminating between the inhibition of MAO A and B. The correlation between the A/B ratio present in different human brain regions and the sensitivity of dopamine oxidation to 10^{-6} M deprenyl was 0.84 (p $<$ 0.001). This suggests that all dopamine oxidation can be accounted for by the joint contribution of MAO A and B and that it is unnecessary to postulate a special form of the enzyme which metabolizes dopamine. In the brain, the striatum has the highest proportion of MAO B, and in several cortical regions, relatively more dopamine is oxidized by MAO A. In other human tissues also the deprenyl sensitivity of dopamine oxidation correlated with the known A/B ratio, the placenta, lung and jejunum having the lowest sensitivity and being the richest in MAO A. K_m values for dopamine for MAO A and B are similar, 130 and 140 μM respectively, so that the proportion oxidized by the two forms should not vary with substrate concentration.

Introduction

Once the dopamine (DA) deficit in Parkinson's disease had been identified (*Ehringer* and *Hornykiewicz*, 1960), one obvious strategy to replenish it was to inhibit the enzyme responsible for its degradation, monoamine oxidase (MAO) and such an approach should have been useful in prolonging the therapeutic effect of L-dopa. An early pharmacological pointer to a successful outcome of this combined regimen was the observation that L-dopa stimulation of reserpinized rats is potentiated by MAO inhibition (*Carlsson et al.*, 1958). However, initial trials of MAO inhibitors with L-dopa in Parkinson's disease (*Birkmayer* and *Hornykiewicz*, 1962), whilst not completely without success, had to be abandoned because of the onset of hypertension (*Birkmayer*, 1966; *Barbeau et al.*, 1962). With the discovery that MAO exists in at least two forms, each with different substrate and inhibitor sensitivity (*Johnston*, 1968), there arose the possibility of selective inhibition without undesirable side effects (*Youdim et al.*, 1971). In 1975, *Birkmayer et al.* first showed that (—)-deprenyl, the selective MAO B inhibitor, is beneficial in Parkinson's disease when added as a supplement to L-dopa therapy. Other studies have confirmed this and the benefit seems to come particularly in prolonging the effect of L-dopa and in alleviating certain types of "on-off" effect (*Lees et al.*, 1977). (—)-Deprenyl also seems singularly free of adverse reactions and is unique amongst the MAO inhibitors in not being associated with the dangerous "cheese effect" (*Elsworth et al.*, 1978).

At the time of Birkmayer's initial trial, it seemed puzzling that a selective MAO B inhibitor should be beneficial in Parkinson's disease, as evidence from rats showed that brain DA is metabolized predominantly by MAO A (*Waldmeier et al.*, 1976). However, in our initial studies (*Glover et al.*, 1977), we found that DA is metabolized predominantly by MAO B in the human striatum, thus providing a rationale for the use of deprenyl in Parkinson's disease and showing once again that the rat cannot automatically be assumed to be a model for man. We report here an extension of our original study. We have examined the metabolism of DA by MAO A and B and its sensitivity to (—)-deprenyl in several human brain regions and tissues.

Materials and Methods

a) *Collection of material:* The jejunal material was obtained from biopsy (*Elsworth et al.*, 1978). Placental tissue was quickly frozen soon after delivery. Platelets were freshly harvested (*Glover et al.*, 1977). All the other tissues were collected at autopsy from 5 subjects (4 male, 1 female) without disease of the nervous system, obtained between 24 and 48 hours after death, up till which time, the bodies had been stored at 4 °C. A sample of each peripheral tissue to be examined was taken as soon as it had been removed from the body and immediately frozen on dry ice where it remained until transferred to permanent storage at −20 °C. Brains were treated similarly except that, before freezing, they were placed in a polystyrene mould on removal from the cranium. This preserved their shape, thus aiding eventual dissection.

b) *Dissection of brains* was by the method of *Owen et al.* (1979), which involves cutting out appropriate areas from thin coronal slices at a low temperature.

c) *Homogenization:* Depending on the particular tissue, homogenates from 10 to 50 mg were prepared in 1 ml 10 mM phosphate buffer at pH 7.4. Either an Ultra Turrax motorized homogenizer or all-glass hand-operated equipment was used.

d) *Assay:* The final concentrations of the three labelled substrates used to determine specific activities were 300 μM for 5-hydroxytryptamine (5-HT) and DA (Radiochemical Centre, Amersham, U.K.) and 125 μM for phenylethylamine (PEA) (New England Nuclear Corp., U.S.A.). The concentrations of DA used to find K_m values ranged from 60 to 600 μM. The linearity of the assay with enzyme concentration was verified. All chosen regions of a single brain were assayed at the same time to ensure that relative activity value comparisons were valid. Samples from different individuals were measured on different days. All MAO activity values are expressed as nmoles oxidized per mg protein per 30 min.

(i) Determination of specific activity: 20 μl of enzyme preparation was added to 100 μl phosphate buffer, pH 7.4, in plastic tubes on ice. 20 μl of either 10^{-2} M deprenyl, for blanks, or water for the sample was then added. After inclusion of 20 μl of radioactive substrate, the rack of tubes was transferred to a shaking bath at 37 °C for 30 min. The reaction was stopped by plunging the tubes into an ice bath and adding 100 μl 2 M citric acid to each. DA and 5-HT were separated from their deaminated products by solvent extraction with 3 ml of a 1 : 1 mixture of ethyl acetate and toluene. PEA extraction was achieved with 3 ml of toluene alone. The organic phase was counted after the addition of 4 ml Instagel (Packard Instruments).

(ii) Determination of deprenyl sensitivity: The procedure above (i) was used except for the following: 20 μl of deprenyl was added to the samples to give a final concentration from 10^{-3} M to 10^{-9} M and prior to addition of substrate, the tubes were preincubated at room temperature for 30 min. To assess the effect of 10^{-6} M deprenyl on DA-oxidizing activity, control tubes with 20 μl water instead of deprenyl were included.

e) *Protein concentration* was measured by the method of *Lowry et al.* (1951).

Results

Fig. 1 shows the effect of different concentrations of (—)-deprenyl on the two forms of the enzyme in human brain material. Samples from different brain regions (cortex and striatum) gave similar results. It will be seen that 10^{-6} M (—)-deprenyl was the most effective at

distinguishing the two forms, inhibiting 5-HT oxidation with a mean
± S.E. of 20 ± 8.5 % and PEA oxidation by 90 ± 2 %.

In Table 1, we show the distribution of 5-HT, PEA and DA-
oxidizing activities in different brain regions and the degree of
inhibition of DA oxidation produced by 10^{-6} M (—)-deprenyl. All the

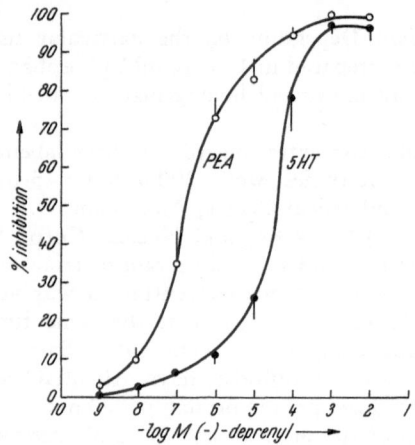

Fig. 1. Selective inhibition by (—)-deprenyl of PEA and 5-HT oxidation in human
striatum. Results represent mean ± S.E. from separate determinations on homogenates of striatum from 6 individuals

Table 1. *5-HT, PEA and DA-oxidizing activities in different regions of
human brain, and inhibition of DA oxidation by 10^{-6} M (—)-deprenyl*

Region	5-HT	PEA	DA	5-HT/ PEA	% inhibition DA oxidation by deprenyl
Accumbens	21.9	21.8	28.5	1.0	83
Caudate	20.2	17.2	29.4	1.2	82
Pallidus	18.0	14.1	21.8	1.3	80
Putamen	16.6	13.1	19.7	1.2	80
Hypothalamus	38.3	22.1	37.2	1.7	70
Amygdala	27.9	14.3	24.8	2.1	73
Precentral cortex	16.7	6.9	13.5	2.4	66
Occipital cortex	20.2	6.0	16.7	3.3	67
Temporal cortex	18.7	8.1	14.5	2.3	65
Frontal cortex	17.6	7.2	12.9	2.4	68
Cerebellar cortex	10.7	4.8	9.6	2.2	63

Results are the means of duplicate assays from 5 brains. Activities are
expressed as nmoles substrate oxidized per mg protein in 30 min.

brains showed a similar pattern. It will be seen that the MAO A/B ratio, is indicated by the ratio of activities using 5-HT and PEA, varied in the different regions and that there was relatively more MAO B in the DA-rich regions of the accumbens and striatum than in the cortical regions. In these regions rich in MAO B, there was also greater sensitivity of DA oxidation to (—)-deprenyl. The correlation between 5-HT/PEA ratio and % inhibition by (—)-deprenyl is 0.84 (p < 0.001). These results would be consistent with DA being a substrate for both MAO A and B but being predominantly metabolized by MAO B, particularly in the DA-rich regions.

To examine the nature of DA oxidation by MAO A and B in more detail we have studied it both in placenta, which contains solely MAO A (*Egashira*, 1976; *Lewinsohn et al.*, in preparation) and in platelets, which contain solely MAO B (*Donnelly* and *Murphy*, 1977). The results are given in Table 2. It will be seen that DA-oxidizing activity was present in both tissues, but that relatively higher activity was associated with PEA (the DA/PEA ratio) than 5-HT (the DA/5-HT ratio). The K_m for DA was similar in both tissues. Some PEA-oxidizing activity was observed in the purely MAO A-containing placenta.

Table 2. *Some characteristics of DA-oxidizing activity in human placenta and platelet*

	Placenta	Platelet
n	3	3
5-HT activity	102	—
DA activity	60.3	7.4
PEA activity	29.8	5.0
DA/5-HT	0.6	—
DA/PEA	—	1.5
% inhibition DA-oxidizing activity by 10^{-6} M deprenyl	23.5	98
K_m, DA (μM)	130	140

MAO activity is expressed as nmoles substrate oxidized per mg protein in 30 min.

In Table 3 we show DA-oxidizing activity and its sensitivity to 10^{-6} M (—)-deprenyl in some other human tissues. Inhibitor sensitivity will be seen to vary widely, the heart being particularly sensitive and the lung insensitive.

Table 3. *DA-oxidizing activity and its inhibition by 10^{-6} M (—)-deprenyl in some peripheral human tissues*

	Activity	% inhibition by deprenyl
Heart	9.1	85
Lung	9.2	22
Kidney	27.5	64
Liver	39.7	60
Jejunum	62.4	34

Results are the means of duplicate assays on tissues from 4 individuals. MAO activity is expressed as nmoles DA oxidized per mg protein in 30 min.

Discussion

These results show that both MAO A and B can metabolize DA in man and that we can relate the degree of (—)-deprenyl sensitivity of DA oxidation to the ratio of MAO A and B present. As K_m values for DA with MAO A and B are very similar, the proportion of DA metabolized by the two forms should not vary with substrate concentration. It has been suggested that there might be an individual MAO for DA (*Youdim*, 1972). Our results provide no evidence for it and we have discovered no organ or brain region where DA oxidation occurs independently of 5-HT or PEA oxidation. It has also been thought possible that the nature of MAO A or B might vary in different tissues of the same individual (*Fowler et al.*, 1978). This remains a possibility but as far as DA oxidation is concerned, the brain enzymes appear to behave in a similar way to those in placenta and platelet. As shown in Table 2, PEA, at the concentration used, is not a very specific substrate for MAO B and the MAO of the placenta, which behaves solely as MAO A in its clorgyline and deprenyl sensitivity, oxidises it to some extent (we now know that benzylamine is considerably more specific than PEA for MAO B [*Lewinsohn et al.*, 1979]). When this contribution of MAO A to PEA-oxidizing activity is taken into consideration in judging the proportion of MAO A and B in brain, the level of DA oxidation in the different regions of the brain can be derived from the sum of contributions of MAO A (calculated by $0.6 \times$ 5-HT activity as in the placenta) and MAO B (calculated as $1.5 \times$ PEA activity in the platelet) (Table 2).

Several peripheral tissues, notably liver, kidney and jejunum, oxidize DA actively, as shown in Table 3. Here also the sensitivity of DA oxidation to deprenyl correlates well with what is known of the proportion of MAO A and B in the various tissues. The lung, found in this investigation to be the least sensitive to deprenyl, has also been shown, in an independent study of ours, to contain MAO A almost exclusively (*Lewinsohn et al.*, 1979). The jejunum also has a high A/B ratio (*Elsworth et al.*, 1978), whereas the heart is relatively rich in MAO B (*Glover et al.*, 1979).

The concentration of (—)-deprenyl which we found to be most selective in human tissues under our *in vitro* conditions is 10^{-6} M. Although some MAO in post-mortem brain material shows anomalous responses to (—)-deprenyl (*Owen et al.*, 1979), no variation in deprenyl sensitivity between individuals was apparent in the present study. (—)-Deprenyl is usually employed clinically at a dose of 10 mg/day and if evenly distributed in a body water mass of 40 kg would give a concentration of 10^{-6} M, suggesting that this dose is the right range for selectivity *in vivo*. However, there are many problems in extrapolating from the *in vivo* to the *in vitro* situation and the *in vivo* effects of this dose need to be determined by independent studies such as by analysis of post-mortem tissues. Preliminary data of *Riederer et al.* (1978) indicate that in subjects treated during life with 10 mg (—)-deprenyl per day, DA oxidizing activity is inhibited 85—90 %, whereas 5-HT-oxdizing activity in the striatum was inhibited by 65 %. The degree of inhibition which affects the *in vivo* function of the enzyme is still unclear. In both rat (*Knoll*, 1978) and man (*Murphy et al.*, 1979) there is some evidence that inhibition of MAO can remain selective on a chronic basis at the right dose. Careful use of MAO inhibitors might, therefore, shed light on the role of the amine substrates of MAO, including DA, in normal function or disease.

A different aspect of the function of MAO B has recently come to light with the realization that it is also important in histamine metabolism. In the brain, where relatively high concentrations are present, histamine is first methylated to *tele*-methylhistamine (TMH) and then oxidized (*Schwartz*, 1977). In both man (*Elsworth et al.*, in preparation) and rat (*Waldmeier et al.*, 1977; *Hough* and *Domino*, 1979) there is new evidence that this oxidation is specifically catalyzed by MAO B. Because histaminase appears to be absent in the brain, the finding assumes particular importance and suggests that (—)-deprenyl, even when used selectively, might control TMH and, perhaps, histamine concentrations as well as those of other and rather more obscure substrates of MAO B such as phenylethanolamine and o-tyramine (*Edwards*, 1978). It will be of interest to see whether deprenyl has any side effects attributable to its effect on histamine metabolism. *Yahr* (1978) mentions a patient whose quiescent peptic ulcer became active on (—)-deprenyl.

12*

It is theoretically possible that, *in vivo*, TMH and DA act as competitive inhibitors for each other and in conditions of high DA concentration, TMH concentration would build up. In this context, it is interesting that PEA has a much higher affinity for MAO ($K_m = 5 \mu M$) than other substrates (*White* and *Wu*, 1975) and if local concentrations of this order were to be reached, then it too would competitively inhibit MAO B, and boost local DA or TMH concentrations accordingly.

Our knowledge of such molecular interactions must at present remain speculative. What is established is that DA is predominantly oxidized by MAO B in human brain. This is particularly true in the DA-rich regions of the striatum, but in the cortical regions also, a substantial proportion is metabolized by this form. It is, therefore, reasonable to expect that deprenyl, at some suitably low selective concentration, would be of benefit in Parkinson's disease.

Acknowledgements

We are grateful to Dr. Rachel Lewinsohn for providing us with some of the tissues used in this investigation and to Prof. J. Knoll and the Chinoin Chemical Co., Budapest, for generous supplies of (—)-deprenyl.

V.G. and J.D.E. are supported by the Parkinson's Disease Society.

References

Barbeau, A., Sourkes, T. L., Murphy, G. F.: Les catécholamines dans la maladie de Parkinson. In: Monoamines et système nerveux central, pp. 247—262. Genève: Georg. 1962.

Birkmayer, W.: Experimentelle Befunde und neue Aspekte bei extrapyramidalen Erkrankungen. Wien. Z. Nervenheilk. *23*, 128—139 (1966).

Birkmayer, W., Hornykiewicz, O.: Der L-Dioxyphenylalanin(L-Dopa-)-Effekt beim Parkinson-Syndrom des Menschen. Arch. Psychiat. Nervenkr. *203*, 560—574 (1962).

Birkmayer, W., Riederer, P., Youdim, M. B. H., Linauer, W.: The potentiation of the anti-kinetic effect after L-dopa treatment by an inhibitor of MAO B, deprenyl. J. Neural Transm. *36*, 303—326 (1975).

Carlsson, A., Lindqvist, M., Magnusson, T., Waldeck, B.: On the presence of 3-hydroxytyramine in brain. Science *127*, 471 (1958).

Donnelly, C. H., Murphy, D. L.: Substrate- and inhibitor-related characteristics of human platelet MAO. Biochem. Pharmacol. *26*, 853—858 (1977).

Edwards, D. J.: Phenylethanolamine is a specific substrate for type B monoamine oxidase. Life Sci. *23*, 1201—1208 (1978).

Egashira, T.: Studies on monoamine oxidase. XVIII. Enzymic properties of placental monoamine oxidase. Jap. J. Pharmacol. *26,* 493—500 (1976).

Ehringer, H., Hornykiewicz, O.: Verteilung von Noradrenalin und Dopamin (3-Hydroxytyramin) im Gehirn des Menschen und ihr Verhalten bei Erkrankungen des extrapyramidalen Systems. Klin. Wschr. *38,* 1236—1239 (1960).

Elsworth, J. D., Glover, V., Reynolds, G. P., Sandler, M., Lees, A. J., Phuapradit, P., Shaw, K., Stern, G. M., Kumar, P.: Deprenyl administration in man: a selective MAO-B inhibitor without the "cheese effect". Psychopharmacology *57,* 33—38 (1978).

Elsworth, J. D., Glover, V., Sandler, M.: tele-Methylhistamine is a monoamine oxidase B substrate in man. (In preparation.)

Fowler, C. J., Callingham, B. A., Mantle, T. J., Tipton, K. F.: Monoamine oxidase A and B: a useful concept? Biochem. Pharmacol. *27,* 97—101 (1978).

Glover, V., Sandler, M., Owen, F., Riley, G. J.: Dopamine is a monoamine oxidase B substrate in man. Nature *265,* 80—81 (1977).

Glover, V., Elsworth, J. D., Sandler, M.: Dopamine oxidation and its inhibition by (—)-deprenyl in human brain and tissues. In: Catecholamines: Basic and Clinical Frontiers (Proc. 4th Catecholamine Symposium, Asilomar, 1978), pp. 201—203. New York: Pergamon Press. 1979.

Hough, L. B., Domino, E. F.: tele-Methylhistamine oxidation by type B monoamine oxidase. J. Pharmacol. exp. Ther. *208,* 422—428 (1979).

Johnston, J. P.: Some observations upon a new inhibitor of monoamine oxidase in brain tissue. Biochem. Pharmacol. *17,* 1285—1297 (1968).

Knoll, J.: The possible mechanisms of action of (—)-deprenyl in Parkinson's disease. J. Neural Transm. *43,* 177—198 (1978).

Lees, A. J., Shaw, K. M., Kohout, L. J., Stern, G. M., Elsworth, J. D., Sandler, M., Youdim, M. B. H.: Deprenyl in Parkinson's disease. Lancet *ii,* 791—795 (1977).

Lewinsohn, R., Glover, V., Sandler, M.: β-Phenylethylamine and benzylamine as substrates for human monoamine oxidase A: a source of some anomalies? Biochem. Pharmacol. (in press, 1979).

Lowry, O. H., Rosebrough, N. J., Farr, A. L., Randall, R. J.: Protein measurement with the Folin phenol reagent. J. biol. Chem. *193,* 265—275 (1951).

Murphy, D. L., Lipper, S., Slater, S., Shilling, D.: Selectivity of clorgyline and pargyline as inhibitors of monoamine oxidases A and B *in vivo* in man. Psychopharmacology *62,* 129—132 (1979).

Owen, F., Cross, A. J., Lofthouse, R., Glover, V.: Distribution and inhibition characteristics of human brain monoamine oxidase. Biochem. Pharmacol. *28,* 1077—1080 (1979).

Riederer, P., Youdim, M. B. H., Rausch, W. D., Birkmayer, W., Jellinger, K., Seemann, D.: On the mode of action of L-deprenyl in the human central nervous system. J. Neural Transm. *43,* 217—226 (1978).

Schwartz, J. C.: Histaminergic mechanisms in brain. Ann. Rev. Pharmacol. Toxicol. *17,* 325—339 (1977).

Waldmeier, P. C., Delini-Stula, A., Maître, L.: Preferential deamination of dopamine by an A type monoamine oxidase in rat brain. Naunyn-Schmiedeberg's Arch. Pharmacol. *292,* 9—14 (1976).

Waldmeier, P. C., Feldtrauer, J.-J., Maître, L.: Methylhistamine: evidence for selective deamination by MAO B in the rat brain *in vivo.* J. Neurochem. *29,* 785—790 (1977).

White, H. L., Wu, J. C.: Multiple binding sites of human brain monoamine oxidase as indicated by substrate competition. J. Neurochem. *25,* 21—26 (1975).

Yahr, M. D.: Overview of present day treatment of Parkinson's disease. J. Neural Transm. *43,* 227—238 (1978).

Youdim, M. B. H.: Multiple forms of monoamine oxidase and their properties. In: Monoamine Oxidases—New Vistas (*Costa, E., Sandler, M.,* eds.), pp. 67—77. New York: Raven Press. 1972.

Youdim, M. B. H., Collins, G. G. S., Sandler, M.: Monoamine oxidase: multiple forms and selective inhibitors. Biochem. J. *121,* 34P—36P (1971).

Authors' address: Prof. *M. Sandler,* Bernhard Baron Memorial Research Laboratories, Queen Charlotte's Maternity Hospital, Goldhawk Road, London W6 OXG, U.K.

Journal of Neural Transmission, Suppl. 16, 173—178 (1980)
© by Springer-Verlag 1980

Dopamine Metabolism in Human Brain: Effects of Monoamine Oxidase Inhibition *in vitro* by (—)Deprenyl and (+) and (—)Tranylcypromine

G. P. Reynolds, P. Riederer, and W.-D. Rausch

Neurochemistry Group, Ludwig Boltzmann-Institute of Clinical Neurobiology,
Lainz-Hospital, Wien, Austria

With 2 Figures

Summary

The effects of the monoamine oxidase inhibitors (—)deprenyl and (+)- and (—)tranylcypromine on dopamine oxidation in human caudate have been investigated. Oxidation of dopamine has been found to exhibit both (—)deprenyl-sensitive and -insensitive components. The tranylcypromine isomers are both more sensitive towards dopamine than 5-hydroxytryptamine oxidation, the (+) isomer being the more effective of the two. These results are discussed in terms of the *in vivo* action of the drugs and their therapeutic value.

Introduction

The neurotransmitter dopamine (DA) is of particular interest in neurological disease since its concentration is greatly diminished in the striatum of patients with Parkinson's disease. This observation has led to effective therapeutic treatment with the DA precursor L-dopa (*Birkmayer* and *Hornykiewicz*, 1962) and, more recently, the supplementation of L-dopa with (—)deprenyl, a monoamine oxidase (MAO) inhibitor (*Birkmayer et al.*, 1975, 1977; *Lees et al.*, 1977). Whether (—)deprenyl exerts its beneficial effect by inhibiting DA oxidation is still unclear, although evidence certainly suggests that in man DA is metabolised by the B form of MAO which is selectively inhibited by (—)deprenyl (*Glover et al.*, 1977).

The research reported here has been carried out in order to further our understanding of the effects of (—)deprenyl on DA metabolism, and to investigate two other inhibitors of DA oxidation, (+)- and (—)tranylcypromine, using samples taken post mortem from human brain.

Methods

Samples of caudate nucleus were taken 6.5 ± 2.5 (S.D.) hours post mortem from 5 subjects (68 ± 3 years) who had not exhibited psychiatric or neurological disorders. The patients had died of heart failure or broncho-pneumonia, and their brains were subjected to routine histopathological examination to rule out any abnormalities affecting brain function. The samples were kept frozen at $-40\,°C$ until analysis of MAO which was carried out using the method of *Tipton* and *Youdim* (1976) with DA, phenylethylamine (PE) or 5-hydroxytryptamine (5-HT) as substrates, used at concentrations of 10^{-3} or 10^{-4} M.

Results and Discussion

Fig. 1 shows a typical inhibition curve of DA oxidation in human caudate using various concentrations of (—)deprenyl. The inflection in the curve, making it almost double-sigmoidal, suggests the presence of a component of DA oxidation which is relatively resistant to (—)deprenyl inhibition. This presumably corresponds to MAO type A, and implies that DA oxidation is not exclusively type B in human caudate. As such a curve is exhibited by a range of DA concentrations between 10^{-5} and 10^{-3} M, we have eliminated the

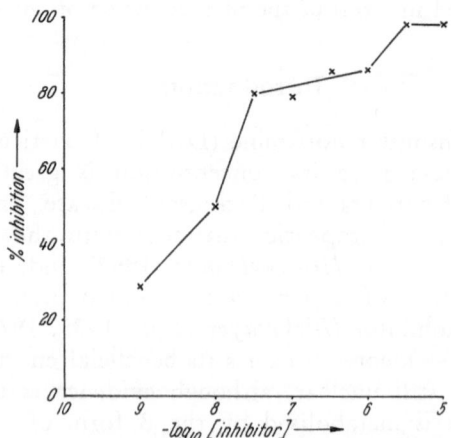

Fig. 1. Inhibition of dopamine oxidation by (—)deprenyl

possibility that high substrate concentration induces type A oxidation, as has been found for PE in rat brain (*Suzuki et al., 1979*).

Other evidence supports these findings. (—)Deprenyl medication in man inhibits platelet MAO (almost exclusively type B) by 100 % (*Elsworth et al., 1978*). Analogously, we have found that this treatment inhibits oxidation of PE (a "pure" B substrate) in the caudate by 97 %, yet only some 88 % of DA-sensitive MAO activity is lost.

Fig. 1 is an inhibition curve taken from a single caudate sample. Other such samples show a similar inhibition pattern, although the level at which the inflection occurs can vary substantially between individuals. Typically this level is at 70—85 % inhibition, although some individuals exhibit particularly low sensitivity towards (—)-deprenyl. This is demonstrated in Table 1, which suggests that those samples with such a low sensitivity also appear to exhibit a low PE oxidising activity (presumably corresponding to MAO-B activity).

Table 1

Patient	Inflection level*	PE oxidation activity (nmol · min^{-1} · mg protein^{-1})
1	21 %	0.23
2	55 %	0.47
3	50 %	0.31
4	73 %	0.81
5	82 %	0.85

* Inhibition of DA oxidation by 10^{-7} M deprenyl

A further interesting observation was found in the study of DA, PE and 5-HT oxidation in caudate taken post mortem from 6 patients. While no significant correlation was found between PE and DA oxidation, DA and 5-HT oxidation were strongly correlated ($r = 0.91$, $p < 0.02$), a finding surprising considering the above data and contrary to the results of *Glover et al.* (1977). A possible explanation of these apparent inconsistencies is the difference in death-to-dissection times which here are only 10—15 % of those of previous reports. Since MAO type A is more sensitive (*White* and *Tansik*, 1979) a loss may occur post mortem leading to an apparent increase in the relative amount of MAO B activity, an effect minimised by short post-mortem times.

These findings have clinical implications in the use of (—)deprenyl in Parkinson's disease. While, as would be expected, PE is increased in human brain after (—)deprenyl treatment (*Reynolds et al., 1978*), it seems questionable whether this would effect an increase in DA, since a substantial fraction of DA oxidising activity still remains. Unfortunately, post-mortem studies of (—)deprenyl treated parkinsonian patients would not necessarily provide an answer since patients dying in the last stages of the disease process have near total loss of dopaminergic function and DA synthesis in the striatum. However, samples from a parkinsonian patient receiving 100 mg/day (—)deprenyl (ten-fold the normal dose) show a significant increase of DA in limbic regions although no increase was found in the striatum (*Riederer et al.*, 1979). This is consistent with increased brain DA in rats found after high dose deprenyl treatment (*Neff* and *Fuentes*, 1976).

Fig. 2 shows the inhibition of human caudate DA oxidation by the two isomers of tranylcypromine. As has been noted in rat brain (*Fuentes et al.*, 1976), the (+) isomer is the better inhibitor, being in this case approximately ten-fold more effective than the (—) isomer. We have noted in addition a selectivity of each form for DA over 5-HT oxidation which, while not as pronounced as that exhibited by (—)deprenyl, is still substantial (Table 2). The results here complement a preliminary *in vivo* study in man, where only the (+) isomer was found to be effective as an MAO inhibitor (*Reynolds et al.*, 1980). As, however, the (—) isomer is a good inhibitor of neuronal amine uptake, like other antidepressants (*Fuentes et al.*, 1976), the rationale behind antidepressant therapy with racemic tranylcypromine ("Parnate") is found to be far from clear. Furthermore, these results suggest that a trial of (+)tranylcypromine as an antiparkinsonian drug in

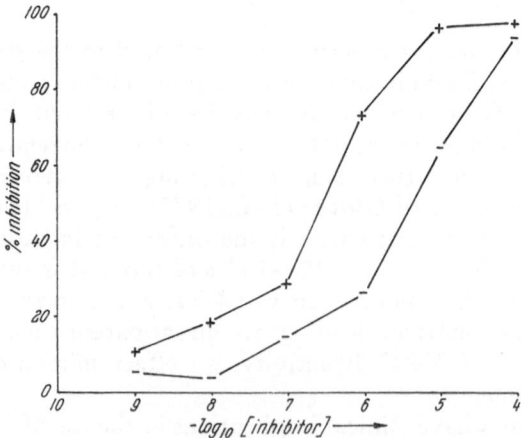

Fig. 2. Inhibition of dopamine oxidation by tranylcypromine isomers.
+ = (+)tranylcypromine, — = (—)tranylcypromine

conjunction with L-dopa should throw light on whether the efficacy of (—)deprenyl in such treatment is indeed due to MAO inhibition or whether another pharmacological effect is involved.

Table 2. *Percentage inhibition of human caudate MAO by 10^{-6} M inhibitor*

	Substrate	
Inhibitor	DA	5-HT
(—)deprenyl	86 %	20 %
(+)tranylcypromine	72 %	35 %
(—)tranylcypromine	27 %	7 %

References

Birkmayer, W., Hornykiewicz, O.: Der L-3, 4-Dioxyphenylalanin- (= Dopa)-Effect bei der Parkinson-Akinese. Wien. klin. Wschr. *73*, 787 (1961).

Birkmayer, W., Riederer, P., Youdim, M. B. H., Linauer, W.: Potentiation of the anti-akinetic effect after L-DOPA treatment by an inhibitor of MAO-B deprenil. J. Neural Transm. *36*, 303—323 (1975).

Birkmayer, W., Riederer, P., Ambrozi, L., Youdim, M. B. H.: Implications of combined treatment with "Madopar" and deprenil in Parkinson's disease: a long term study. Lancet *I*, 434—443 (1977).

Elsworth, J. D., Glover, V., Reynolds, G. P., Sandler, M., Lees, A. J., Phuapradit, P., Shaw, K. M., Stern, G. M., Kumar, P.: Deprenyl administration in man: A selective monoamine oxidase B inhibitor without the "cheese effect". Psychopharmacol. *57*, 33—38 (1978).

Fuentes, J. A., Oleshansky, M. A., Neff, N. H.: Comparison of the apparent antidepressant activity of (—) and (+) tranylcypromine in an animal model. Biochem. Pharmacol. *25*, 801—804 (1976).

Glover, V., Sandler, M., Owen, F., Riley, G. J.: Dopamine is a monoamine oxidase B substrate in man. Nature *265*, 80—81 (1977).

Lees, A. J., Shaw, K. M., Kohout, L. J., Stern, G. M., Elsworth, J. D., Sandler, M., Youdim, M. B. H.: Deprenyl in Parkinson's disease. Lancet *II*, 791—796 (1977).

Neff, N. H., Fuentes, J. A.: The use of selective monoamine oxidase inhibitor drugs for evaluating pharmacological and physiological mechanisms. In: Monoamine oxidase and its inhibition (*Wolstenholme, G. E. W., Knight, J.,* eds), pp. 163—173. Amsterdam: Elsevier. 1976.

Reynolds, G. P., Riederer, P., Sandler, M., Jellinger, K., Seemann, D.: Amphetamine and 2-phenylethylamine in post-mortem parkinsonian brain after (—)deprenyl administration. J. Neural Transm. *43*, 271—277 (1978).

Reynolds, G. P., Rausch, W.-D., Riederer, P.: Effects of tranylcypromine stereoisomers on monoamine oxidation in man. Brit. J. Clin. Pharmacol. (1980, in press).

Riederer, P., Reynolds, G. P., Birkmayer, W., Youdim, M. B. H., Jellinger, K.: (—)Deprenyl has a band of selectivity for therapeutic action. In: Proceedings of the 3rd Hungarian Pharmacological Congress, 1979.

Suzuki, O., Katsumata, Y., Oya, M., Matsumoto, T.: Effect of β-phenylethylamine concentration on its substrate specificity for type A and type B monoamine oxidase. Biochem. Pharmacol. 28, 953—956 (1979).

Tipton, K., Youdim, M. B. H.: Assay of monoamine oxidase. In: Monoamine oxidase and its inhibition (*Wolstenholme, G. E. W., Knight, J.*, eds.), pp. 393—403. Amsterdam: Elsevier. 1976.

White, H., Tansik, R. L.: Characterisation of multiple substrate binding sites of MAO. In: Symposium on Monoamine oxidase structure, function and altered functions. Midland, Michigan, 1979.

Authors' address: Doz. Dr. *P. Riederer,* Neurochemistry Group, Ludwig Boltzmann-Institute of Clinical Neurobiology, Lainz-Hospital, Wolkersbergenstrasse 1, A-1130 Wien, Austria.

Journal of Neural Transmission, Suppl. 16, 179—185 (1980)
© by Springer-Verlag 1980

Unilateral Parkinson's Disease and Contralateral Tardive Dyskinesia: A Unique Case with Successful Therapy That May Explain the Pathophysiology of These Two Disorders

S. Fahn and R. Mayeux

Department of Neurology, College of Physicians and Surgeons, Columbia University, and The Neurological Institute of New York, New York, U.S.A.

Summary

A unique case is reported of a patient with right-sided Parkinson's disease and left-sided tardive dyskinesia. This situation occurred because the patient's parkinsonian tremor was treated with antipsychotic drugs. After several months she developed tardive dyskinesia on the left side of the body. Successful treatment was achieved nine years later, using dopamine-depleting drugs (combination reserpine and alpha-methylparatyrosine) to suppress the tardive dyskinesia and trihexyphenidyl to reduce the parkinsonism. Control of the symptoms was complicated when parkinsonism symptoms later increased on the right and developed on the left, due to the dopamine-depleting drugs. A small amount of carbidopa/levodopa restored the proper balance of symptoms, effectively reducing the parkinsonism while not aggravating the tardive dyskinesia.

This unique case provides insight into the pathogenesis of Parkinson's disease, the pathogenesis of tardive dyskinesia, their successful therapeutic approaches, and possibly the effect of drugs in blocking the progression of Parkinson's disease.

Introduction

Tardive dyskinesia (TD) is a drug-induced disorder characterized by repetitive (stereotypic) choreic movements, particularly in the oral region (oral-lingual-buccal dyskinesia), but may involve other parts of the body as well (body rocking, respiratory tics, piano playing fingers and toes, marching in place). It is an iatrogenic disorder associated with chronic usage of antipsychotic drugs which act as blockers of postsynaptic dopamine receptors. The incidence is higher in women than men, and the elderly seem particularly affected (*Crane*, 1968). Several mechanisms have been proposed, but the most popular concept is that the postsynaptic dopamine receptor in striatum has become supersensitive and responds excessively to dopamine that reaches it to produce the involuntary movements (*Klawans*, 1973; *Tarsy* and *Baldessarini*, 1976). Many patients with TD have tardive akathisia as well, and this symptom is usually more distressing than the involuntary movements (*Fahn*, 1978 a; *Forrest* and *Fahn*, 1979). The cerebral locus for this persistent akathisia is a matter of conjecture, but conceivably, dopamine receptor supersensitivity in the limbic system may be involved. Suppression of TD can be accomplished by increasing the dosage of antipsychotic drugs or by using dopamine depleting agents, with the likelihood of inducing parkinsonism.

An unusual clinical situation presented itself to us with a patient who had features of parkinsonism on the right side of the body and TD on the left side. Not only is this case unique, but the question of how to treat this condition presented a dilemma since drugs that control parkinsonism (*e.g.* levodopa) could increase the TD syndrome on the left side, whereas drugs that control TD (antidopaminergic agents) could aggravate the right hemiparkinsonism. A successful solution was obtained based on consideration of the pathogenesis of these two conditions and the mechanisms of drug actions.

Case Report

At about the age of 64, this woman developed a tremor at rest in her right hand and complained of nervousness. She was treated with perphenazine, 6 mg/day, and amitriptyline, 30 mg/day, without improvement. These medications were continued for at least five months, but the exact duration is not known. At age 65, persistent irregular involuntary movements of the left arm and leg were noted. At age 66, another physician noticed rhythmic involuntary movements of the mouth. Amantadine, 200 mg/day, and diazepam, 40 mg/day, were of no benefit, and were discontinued. She gradually developed increasing stiffness of the right arm and leg and worsening of the oral dyskinesia. Levodopa, 2 gm/day, increased the oral dyskinesia and the "chorea-like" movements of the left arm and leg. It was discontinued after six months and haloperidol, 1.5 mg/day, was then given; this reduced the dyskinesia on the face and left arm or legs, but shuffling gait and cogwheel rigidity were now observed. Haloperidol was increased to 3.5 mg/day and trihexyphenidyl, 4 mg/day, was added, but the amplitude of the right hand tremor increased. Haloperidol was discontinued after three months of use because respiratory gasps and snorting were noted. All medications were discontinued at this point and the involuntary movements on the left became worse. A brief trial of reserpine, 0.75 mg/day, produced no improvement.

At age 67, while not on medications she continued to complain of respiratory gasping, snorting, swallowing difficulty, and involuntary movements of the left arm and leg. Chlorpromazine, 100 mg/day, resulted in improvement of these involuntary movements for several months; however, rigidity, and more severe tremor on the right occurred gradually. Benztropine, 6 mg/day, was added but without improvement. She continued to take chlorpromazine and at age 69 phenytoin, 300 mg/day, was added. The combination of the medications was considered successful in reducing the tremor and dyskinetic movements. Four years later (age 73) the involuntary movements reappeared in the left arm and leg. She was unable to eat, stand, walk or care for herself. Carbidopa/levodopa was tried briefly, but made her worse. At age 74 she was hospitalized. Periodic twitching and jerking movements of the left hand and arm, violent movements of the left leg, and facial grimacing were described. The resting tremor on the right hand persisted. Chlorpromazine and phenytoin were discontinued. A trial of propranolol, 40 mg/day, was given, but this did not improve the tremor. Reserpine, 1 mg/day, was prescribed but discontinued because of headache, somnolence, and lightheadedness. Trifluperazine, 8 mg/day, resulted in remarkable improvement for approximately two weeks, but then all of her symptoms returned. At that time trifluperazine was discontinued and she was transferred to the Neurological Institute for admission. She complained of right sided resting tremor, slowness and stiffness, with severe, often violent involuntary movements of the left arm, leg and face.

Examination revealed an elderly woman with thinning of her hair. She was awake, alert, attentive and somewhat dysarthric, but without impairment of speech, memory or intellect. The cranial nerves were normal except for repetitive chewing movements. There was moderate to severe cogwheel rigidity in the arms and legs, more severe on the right than on the left. A rhythmic 5/sec tremor was noted in the right leg, and a less prominent tremor was noted in the right arm. The tremor became more pronounced when the patient walked. On the left, irregular and regular movements were present in three distinct locations. First, repetitive protrusion of the tongue and movements of the left side of the mouth were present. Second, there was continuous flexion and extension of the first two digits of the left hand in a "snapping-like" movement against the thumb. Third, a similar repetitive flexion-extension dyskinesia was noted distally in the left leg, most pronounced at the ankle but also present at the knee. These movements worsened with anxiety and were absent during sleep. Sensation and coordination were normal. The tremor of the right hand and leg diminished with intention but worsened on the left. The posture was slightly stooped. Adduction of both arms and flexion at the elbow and wrists was present. Postural stability was poor. Tendon reflexes were normal and a positive glabellar reflex was present.

Lumbar puncture, computed tomography of the head, blood chemistries were all normal. Methscopolamine, 1 mg, followed by physostigmine, 2 mg, intravenously resulted in a marked increase in the amplitude of the tremor on the right side; however, a slight decrement of the involuntary movements on the left was noted. Later, benztropine, 1.5 mg, intravenously produced a remarkable subjective feeling of improvement and a lessening of the amplitude of right sided tremor.

She was then treated with trihexyphenidyl, 4 mg, and had less rigidity and tremor and mobility of the right arm and leg. Reserpine was added at a dose of 0.4 mg/day, and gradually increased to 5 mg/day over a $1^1/_2$ week interval. This resulted in 80 % improvement of the buccofacial dyskinesia as well as a 60 % improvement of the dyskinesia on the left. The addition of alpha-methylparatyrosine (AMPT), 250 mg/day, resulted in almost complete elimination of the involuntary movements of the face and left side. The patient was ambulatory and discharged. She was able to live alone. She initially noted drowsiness with AMPT and the dosage was lowered to 125 mg on alternate days. She was maintained on the combination of trihexyphenidyl 4 mg, reserpine 4.4 mg and AMPT 250 mg/125 mg. Three months later she developed a slight increase in rigidity on the right and difficulty swallowing. Carbidopa/levodopa, 5/50 mg t.i.d., remarkably improved her mobility, rigidity and tremor. It did not induce worsening of the dyskinesia of the left arm and leg.

At the present time, at age 75, one year after beginning the above therapy, she lives independently of her family. Occasional assistance is required for some chores and she is unable to operate an automobile. She does have difficulty swallowing with rare choking. Her thinking and memory are clear with no evidence of intellectual impairment. She is able to prepare her own meals although slowly. Current examination reveals a slight buccofacial dyskinesia (0.5/4) and the dyskinesia of the left leg has also improved (0.5/4); however, a moderate dyskinesia of the left hand has persisted (2/4). On the right there is mild rigidity (1/4) in the arm and leg and no tremor is noted. Her gait shows mild shuffling but is not bradykinetic, and her postural stability is still somewhat impaired.

Discussion

1. Striatal Mechanisms in Parkinson's Disease (PD)

The initial defect in this patient's clinical problem was right hemiparkinsonism. Based upon current understanding, this would be due to loss of left nigrostriatal neurons with resulting depletion of dopamine-containing nerve terminals in striatum (*Hornykiewicz*, 1972). Most patients with PD begin with unilateral involvement which may be limited to that one side for a number of years before the other side is involved (*Fahn* and *Duffy*, 1977). In rare cases, the disease may remain unilateral for more than ten years (*Scott et al.*, 1970). With presynaptic dopamine depletion in PD, supersensitivity of the postsynaptic dopamine receptor normally occurs (*Ungerstedt*, 1971). The lack of endogenous dopamine in the striatum would explain why postsynaptic supersensitivity fails to result in chorea;

however, when dopamine is supplied by exogenous levodopa, chorea is a common consequence in patients with parkinsonism.

2. Why Was TD Unilateral and Not Bilateral?

Our patient should have left-sided striatal dopamine deficiency with supersensitive left-sided postsynaptic dopamine receptors. The chronic administration of antipsychotic drugs would now result in supersensitive postsynaptic dopamine receptors in the right striatum as well (*Klawans*, 1973; *Tarsy* and *Baldessarini*, 1976). But the presence of presynaptic dopamine in the right striatum due to intact nigrostriatal neurons, with some of this dopamine penetrating the receptor blockade, would account for the left-sided TD. Thus, we can envision how our patient can have both unilateral PD and contralateral TD. Why didn't the right side of the body also develop TD? The best explanation is that this disorder requires an intact (or excess?) (*Fahn*, 1976) concentration or turnover of dopamine in the nigrostriatal terminals. In PD, there is a deficiency of striatal dopamine, and this condition would preclude the development of TD. In fact, we are not aware of any report of a case of TD developing in a patient having PD.

3. Therapeutic Dilemmas and Solutions

Of the two syndromes, right-sided PD and left-sided TD, in our patient, the more distressing problem was TD, and its control was our first aim of therapy. It was reasoned that dopamine-depleting drugs which act presynaptically, while reducing TD, may aggravate PD only slightly since the presynaptic dopamine neurons in the striatum are predominantly absent, and there is little anatomical substrate remaining to be affected by such drugs. Only with high dosage reserpine with AMPT, was the right hemiparkinsonism increased. In this situation the left-sided TD was replaced by parkinsonism as well. Combination reserpine/AMPT had been used successfully in other patients with TD, and appears to be a most powerful regimen to suppress TD and akathisia (*Fahn*, 1978 b).

The above results are thus compatible with the existing hypotheses of PD being due to a deficiency of presynaptic dopamine and TD being due to supersensitive postsynaptic dopamine receptors. The results do not exclude this possibility that excessive dopamine synthesis presynaptically could also play a role in the pathogenesis of TD, however.

The question of how best to treat the right hemiparkinsonism was then considered. It was believed that increasing striatal dopamine by treating with levodopa would aggravate the TD syndrome (*Klawans* and *McKendall*, 1971), so this approach was avoided initially. The use of anticholinergics only rarely induces chorea (*Fahn* and *David*, 1972; *Birket-Smith*, 1974). Therefore trihexyphenidyl was our initial choice, which had the desired effect of reducing right-sided PD without worsening TD. This was maintained in the presence of dopamine-depleting drugs, and supports the concept that anticholinergics act at the next neuron downstream to produce its antiparkinson effect. However, with high dosage reserpine combined with AMPT, there was an increase of the right hemiparkinsonism and signs of parkinsonism replaced TD on the left side. This complication was corrected with the addition of a small amount of carbidopa/levodopa, a technique used successfully in another patient with TD treated with reserpine/AMPT and in whom it was difficult to titrate the dosages to avoid drug-induced parkinsonism as an adverse effect.

4. Failure of PD To Become Generalized

Finally, wo should discuss the question as to why parkinsonism did not spread to involve loss of the right nigrostriatal neurons. Although PD usually begins on one side of the body (*Hoehn* and *Yahr*, 1967), it is rare for the disease not to become bilateral within ten years (*Scott et al.*, 1970). Our patient has had parkinsonism symptoms for 11 years. Several possible answers suggest themselves: (1) Our patient had one of the rare types of benign hemiparkinsonism, *i.e.* PD that did not become bilateral; (2) she did not have classical PD, but had some other form of parkinsonism, possibly secondary to a focal left hemisphere lesion; (3) the use of antipsychotic drugs somehow prevented or delayed the pathogenesis of nigrostriatal neuron loss. There is no evidence of secondary parkinsonism in our patient, and the second possibility seems unlikely. The third possibility is the most intriguing. If true, it may suggest clues (1) to the pathogenesis of the loss of nigrostriatal neuron in PD, and (2) to a therapeutic approach to prevent further progression of the disease process. The induction of supersensitive DA receptors by antipsychotic drugs should not be a factor in preventing further nigrostriatal neuronal loss, since such supersensitivity occurs in PD and the disease continues to progress. We should consider the possibility that antipsychotic drugs have an action on the nigrostriatal neuron directly, and this action antagonizes the degeneration of the neuron. Should we try to prevent PD from progressing by treating patients in their early stages, especially if already bilateral, with antipsychotic drugs? That question is intriguing and needs to be answered.

References

Birket-Smith, E.: Abnormal involuntary movements induced by anticholinergic medication. Acta Neurol. Scand. *50*, 801—811 (1974).

Crane, G. E.: Tardive dyskinesia in patients treated with major neuroleptics: A review of the literature. Am. J. Psychiat. *124*, suppl., 40—48 (1968).

Fahn, S.: Medical treatment of movement disorders. In: Neurological Reviews 1976, pp. 72—106. Minneapolis: American Academy of Neurology. 1976.

Fahn, S.: Akathisia in tardive dyskinesia. New Engl. J. Med. *299*, 202 to 203 (1978 a).

Fahn, S.: Treatment of tardive dyskinesia with combined reserpine and alpha-methyltyrosine. Trans. Am. Neurol. Assoc. *103*, 100—103 (1978 b).

Fahn, S., David, E.: Oral-facial-lingual dyskinesia due to anticholinergic medication. Trans. Am. Neurol. Assoc. *97*, 277—279 (1972).

Fahn, S., Duffy, P.: Parkinson's disease. In: Scientific Approaches to Clinical Neurology (*Goldensohn, E. S., Appel, S. H.*, eds.), pp. 1119—1158. Philadelphia: Lea and Febiger. 1977.

Forrest, D. V., Fahn, S.: Tardive dysphrenia and subjective akathisia. J. Clin. Psychiat. *40*, 206 (1979).

Hornykiewicz, O.: Dopamine and extrapyramidal motor function and dysfunction. Res. Publ. Assoc. Res. Nerv. Ment. Dis. *50*, 390—412 (1972).

Hoehn, M. M., Yahr, M. D.: Parkinsonism: onset, progression, and mortality. Neurology *17*, 427—442 (1967).

Klawans, H. L.: The pharmacology of tardive dyskinesia. Am. J. Psychiat. *130*, 82—86 (1973).

Klawans, H. L., McKendall, R. R.: Observations on the effect of levodopa on tardive lingual-facial-buccal dyskinesia. J. Neurol. Sci. *14*, 189—192 (1971).

Scott, R. M., Brody, J. A., Schwab, R. S., Cooper, I. S.: Progression of unilateral tremor and rigidity in Parkinson's disease. Neurology *20*, 710—714 (1970).

Tarsy, D., Baldessarini, R. J.: The tardive dyskinesia syndrome. Clin. Neuropharmacol. *1*, 29—61 (1976).

Ungerstedt, U.: Mechanism of action of L-dopa studied in an experimental Parkinson model. In: Monoamines Noyaux Gris Centraux et Syndrome de Parkinson (*de Ajuriaguerra, J., Gauthier, G.*, eds.), pp. 165—170 (Proceedings of the IVth Bel-Air Symposium). Geneva: Georg and Cie. 1971.

Authors' address: *S. Fahn*, M.D., Department of Neurology, College of Physicians and Surgeons, Columbia University, 630 West 168th Street, New York, NY 10032, U.S.A.

Journal of Neural Transmission, Suppl. 16, 187—193 (1980)
© by Springer-Verlag 1980

Lecithin in Parkinson's Disease

A. Barbeau

Department of Neurobiology, Clinical Research Institute of Montreal, Quebec,
Canada

Summary

Pathological and biochemical evidence reviewed favours the hypothesis that the dementia seen in Parkinson's disease, particularly after long-term levodopa therapy, is akin to Alzheimer's disease. We postulate, in late Parkinson's disease, the development of a relative cholinergic deficiency due to the accelerated process of aging and the presence of neurofibrillary tangles (with choline acetyl transferase deficiency). This process would be enhanced by the imbalance in favour of dopaminergic predominance caused by chronic levodopa therapy, and would partially explain the increase in dementia. As a test of this hypothesis we have given 10 levodopa-treated parkinsonian patients with dementia, a regimen of lecithin (average 20 gms/day). A clear improvement in Kohs block design test of constructive ability was noted with a decrease in the toxic symptoms of confusion, hallucinations and nightmares. In another study lecithin produced a decrease in levodopa-induced abnormal movements, but at the expense of motor performance. These preliminary investigations indicate that the progressive dementia of Parkinson's disease may not be irreversible.

The treatment of degenerative disorders of the central nervous system has only recently been undertaken in a systematic fashion. With the use of levodopa in Parkinson's disease (*Barbeau*, 1961; *Birkmayer* and *Hornykiewicz*, 1961) it was demonstrated that some heretofore irreversible symptoms, such as akinesia, could be significantly modified using the principle of replacement therapy of the missing neurotransmitter with its natural precursor. Subsequently *Cohen* and *Wurtman* (1975) clearly indicated that the brain levels of some of the neurotransmitters could also be controlled through variations in the dietary intake of these precursors.

Many of the symptoms of extrapyramidal disorders are the result of a functional imbalance between specific neurotransmitters (*Barbeau*, 1962). Thus the akinesia of Parkinson's disease is due to the specific deficiency of nigrostriatal dopamine, while the other symptoms involve some form of central cholinergic predominance. This, of course, has been the basis of the standard therapy of Parkinson's disease with anticholinergic drugs and later of the replacement therapy with levodopa alone or combined with a peripheral DOPA-decarboxylase inhibitor.

With long-term use of levodopa, a number of side-effects have been seen: abnormal involuntary movements, oscillations in performance, progressive unresponsiveness and increasing dementia (*Barbeau*, (1974, 1976). The analysis of the pathogenesis of these phenomena has revealed changes in receptor sensitivity, pathological and radiological evidence of progressive atrophy and biochemical changes seen normally in the process of aging. Contrary to what was heretofore believed, the primary process of aging is not a generalized or diffuse phenomenon, but appears localized and sometimes restricted to some neuronal complexes. The following areas are more susceptible: the substantia nigra, the locus coeruleus, the striatum, the centre median of the thalamus, the dorsal nucleus of the vagus, the inferior olive and dentate nucleus, and the basal nucleus of Reichert. It is of interest that many of these areas are pigmented and are involved in the synthesis and regulation of specific monoaminergic fiber systems. If one correlates this localized damage with postulated physiological functions, one can understand the "extrapyramidal" clinical manifestations of old age as well as many of the symptoms one observes in parkinsonian patients after many years of treatment. For example, damage to the olive and dentate nucleus could explain the increase in tremor and instability. The centre median and locus coeruleus are known to be implicated in sleep regulation. Involvement of the basal nucleus of Reichert is believed by some to be related to a slowing of thinking, a delay and reduction of emotional reactions, a failure of distributive attention, and finally to a difficulty in decision making.

Many of the biochemical changes found in the aging brain closely parallel what is also found in Parkinson's disease (*Samoroyski*, 1977). Changes have been seen in enzymes and neurotransmitters, as well as in the functions of the hypothalamus. Lowered levels of homovanillic acid (HVA) and 5-hydroxyindoleacetic acid (5-HIAA) in the lumbar cerebrospinal fluid (CSF) have been found in Parkinson's disease and in the senile or presenile forms of dementia, where the more severe the dementia, the lower the levels of the acids (*Gottfries*, *Gottfries*, and *Roos*, 1970). More evidence of the involvement of dopamine metabolism in the process of old age can be obtained by the determination of enzymes in the blood and in brain tissues. The first studies of enzymes in aged brain are those of *McGeer, Fibiger, McGeer,* and *Wickson* (1971). These authors demonstrated that tyrosine-hydroxylase activity in the caudate showed a sharp drop in aged rats and that this drop was both more pronounced and more clearly correlated with age than were changes in other enzymes. Dopamine-β-hydroxylase, which catalyses the last step in noradrenaline biosynthesis, increases with age in human serum (*Freedman et al.,* 1972). In general it can be said that most synthesizing enzymes (TH, DOPA-decarboxylase, GAD) are decreased with age while catabolizing enzymes (monoamine oxidase, catechol-O-methyltransferase) tend to increase. Three main areas seem to be preferentially affected: the caudate-putamen, the substantia nigra and the nucleus accumbens; all three areas are rich in dopamine. The decreased capacity to synthesize catecholamines, coupled with increasing MAO activity, could explain the decreased sensitivity to amphetamine reported in aged animals, the changes in dopamine receptor sensitivity in brain and retina and possibly the loss of responsiveness to L-DOPA noted in Parkinson's disease after long-term treatment. On the other hand, the progressive encroachment upon the noradrenergic systems (locus coeruleus), whose distribution pattern is less selective but is diffuse to nearly all parts of the brain, will definitely affect the "drive" component of motor and mental behaviour. Finally recent studies on the biochemistry of dementia have demonstrated that choline acetyl transferase (CAT) is decreased in most forms of Alzheimer's disease (*Davies* and *Maloney,* 1976) along with the presence of neurofibrillary tangles (paired helical filaments).

It is thus of great interest to note that, as Parkinson's disease progresses, there is evidence of advanced cortical atrophy and ventricular enlargement (*Schneider et al.,* 1979 a; *Schneider et al.,* 1979 b; *Becker et al.,* 1979) similar to what occurs, later, in aging (*Earnest et al.,* 1979). A most intriguing paper by *Hakim* and *Mathieson* (1979) indicates that the average brain weight in Parkinson's disease was 1.281 gm as compared to 1.365 gm for sex- and aged-matched controls. Plaques, neurofibrillary tangles, granulovacuolar degeneration and cortical cell loss were present in all but one of the 34 parkinsonian brains studied, a percentage markedly superior to that in control brains. 56 percent of the parkinsonians in that study were clinically demented, as compared to 6 % of the control matched population.

In summary, from our review, it appears that parkinsonian patients suffer from a form of premature aging accompanied by cortical atrophy, ventricular hypertrophy and the pathologic and clinical findings of Alzheimer's disease. It is therefore warranted to postulate that parkinsonian patients in the normal course of their evolution, will develop a relative cholinergic deficiency. This should be made worse by the tipping of the balance towards dopaminergic preponderance after long-term levodopa therapy. It is thus possible that both the symptoms of dyskinesias and of dementia could be related to such relative cholinergic insufficiency.

In order to test this hypothesis, and possibly to modify the acquired symptoms, we attempted to use a replacement therapy with the possible precursor lecithin, as reviewed in detail in another paper (*Barbeau*, 1978). This approach, of course, is based upon the important studies of *Wurtman* and coworkers (*Cohen* and *Wurtman*, 1975, 1976; *Wurtman, Hirsch*, and *Growdon*, 1977) which showed that the administration of choline chloride causes a sequential increase in serum choline, brain choline, and brain acetylcholine levels. The increase in acetylcholine occurs within presynaptic terminals and is followed by biochemical changes within postsynaptic cells that have a cholinergic innervation. More recent studies (*Wurtman et al.*, 1977) have shown that oral lecithin (phosphatidyl choline) is more effective in raising human serum choline levels than the equivalent quantity of choline chloride. This rise persists much longer after lecithin administration. Two pilot uncontrolled studies were carried out, each on 10 parkinsonian patients, in order to test the effect of lecithin on abnormal involuntary movements and on late appearing dementia. Lecithin granules (Sigma Chemical Company, St. Louis, Missouri) were given in daily doses varying from 3.1 to 30.0 grams, generally in orange juice or chocolate milk. Divided doses were preferred for higher levels. Movements in the hyperkinetic disorders were evaluated from five-minute film strips by two independent observers.

In the 10 parkinsonian patients who were experiencing considerable discomfort because of severe abnormal involuntary movements induced by levodopa, lecithin produced a marked reduction in the number and severity of the dyskinesia (Table 1). Unfortunately there was also a concomitant reduction in the motor performance score of the patients, explained by a return of some degree of rigidity and akinesia. None of the patients were receiving anticholinergic drugs concurrently.

In the 10 parkinsonian patients who were demented after an average of 5.6 years on levodopa therapy (with Sinemet®, average dose 800 mg of levodopa equivalent), lecithin over a period of 3 months was able (Table 2) to improve the performance as measured on the Kohs block design test. Patients and their families noted a

Table 1. *Lecithin in the levodopa-induced abnormal involuntary movements (A.I.M.) of Parkinson's disease (N = 10)*

1. Average daily dose (Lecithin)	20.2 ± 5.8 gms
2. A.I.M. Score	
a) before treatment (Lecithin)	27.0 ± 5.1
b) during treatment	11.1 ± 1.8
3. Motor performance score	
a) before treatment (Lecithin)	527 ± 33
b) at end of treatment	486 ± 28

Table 2. *Kohs block design test before and after Lecithin in levodopa-treated parkinsonian patients (N = 10)*

1. Average daily dose (Lecithin)	19.8 ± 4.6 gms
2. Kohs block design test	
a) before treatment (Lecithin)	22.8 ± 1.9
b) at end of treatment	38.4 ± 3.2
3. Motor performance score	
a) before treatment (Lecithin)	548 ± 52
b) at end of treatment	501 ± 38

significant decrease in periods of confusion, in visual hallucinations, in nightmares, in attitude towards their environment and, less frequently, in recent memory. Four of the 10 patients stated that "their mind was much clearer". It should be stressed that the dose of levodopa equivalent was kept constant during the period of observation.

These studies should be accepted for what they are: pilot investigations of a new hypothesis. The generally positive responses obtained, particularly on constructive performance, as measured by the Kohs block design test, constitute preliminary evidence in favour of the presence of a relative cholinergic deficiency in demented, long-term levodopa-treated, parkinsonian patients and offer the hope that this form of replacement therapy could be advantageous to counter some of the mental effects of advancing age and of long-term levodopa therapy in Parkinson's disease. Controlled, cross-over studies are now being undertaken.

Acknowledgements

The studies reported in this paper were supported in part by grants from the Medical Research Council of Canada (MA 4938), the W. Garfield

Weston Foundation and the Seymour E. Clonick Memorial Fund of the United Parkinson Foundation.

References

Barbeau, A.: Biochemistry of Parkinson's disease. Excerpta Medica Int. Congr. Ser. *38*, 152—153 (1961).

Barbeau, A.: The pathogenesis of Parkinson's disease: a new hypothesis. Can. Med. Ass. J. *87*, 802—807 (1962).

Barbeau, A.: The clinical physiology of side-effects in long-term L-DOPA therapy. In: Advances in Neurology, Vol. 5 (*McDowell, F. H., Barbeau, A.,* eds.), pp. 347—365. New York: Raven Press. 1979.

Barbeau, A.: Neurological and psychiatric side-effects of L-DOPA. In: Int. Encyclop. of Pharmacol. and Therap., Sect. 25 (*Hornykiewicz, O.,* ed.), Vol. 1, pp. 475—494 (1976).

Barbeau, A.: Emerging treatments: replacement therapy with choline or lecithin in neurological diseases. Can. J. Neurol. Sci. *5*, 157—160 (1978).

Becker, H., Schneider, E., Hacker, H., Fischer, P. A.: Cerebral atrophy in Parkinson's disease—represented in CT. Arch. Psychiat. Nervenkr. *227*, 81—88 (1979).

Birkmayer, W., Hornykiewicz, O.: Der L-Dioxyphenylalanin(DOPA-)-Effekt bei der Parkinson-Akinese. Wien. klin. Wschr. *73*, 787—788 (1961).

Cohen, E. L., Wurtman, R. J.: Brain acetylcholine: increase after systemic choline administration. Life Sci. *16*, 1095—1102 (1975).

Cohen, E. L., Wurtman, R. J.: Brain acetylcholine: control by dietary choline. Science *191*, 561—562 (1976).

Davies, S. P., Maloney, A. J. F.: Selective loss of central cholinergic neurons in Alzheimer's disease. Lancet 2, 1403 (1976).

Earnest, M. P., Heaton, R. K., Wilkinson, W. E., Manke, W. F.: Cortical atrophy, ventricular enlargement and intellectual impairment in the aged. Neurology (Minneap.) *29*, 1138—1143 (1979).

Freedman, L. S., Ohuchi, T., Goldstein, M., Axelrod, F., Fish, I., Dancis, J.: Changes in human serum dopamine-β-hydroxylase activity with age. Nature (London) *236*, 310—311 (1972).

Gottfries, C. G., Gottfries, I., Ross, B. E.: Homovanillic acid and 5-hydroxyindole acetic acid in cerebrospinal fluid related to rated mental and motor impairment in senile and presenile dementia. Acta Psychiat. Neurol. Scand. *46*, 99—103 (1970).

Hakim, A. M., Mathieson, G.: Dementia in Parkinson's disease: a neuropathologic study. Neurology (Minneap.) *29*, 1209—1214 (1979).

McGeer, E. G., Fibiger, H. C., McGeer, P. L., Wickson, V.: Aging and brain enzymes. Experim. Gerontology *6*, 391—396 (1971).

Samoroyski, T.: Central neurotransmitter substances and aging: a review. J. Am. Geriat. Soc. *25,* 337—348 (1977).

Schneider, E., Becker, H., Fischer, P. A., Graw, H., Jacobi, P., Brinkmann, R.: The course of brain atrophy in Parkinson's disease. Arch. Psychiat. Nervenkr. *227,* 89—95 (1979 a).

Schneider, E., Fischer, P. A., Jacobi, P., Becker, H., Hacker, H.: The significance of cerebral atrophy for the symptomatology of Parkinson's disease. J. neurol. Sci. *42,* 187—197 (1979 b).

Wurtman, R. J., Hirsch, M. J., Growdon, J. H.: Lecithin consumption raises serum-free choline levels. Lancet *2,* 68—69 (1977).

Author's address: Dr. *A. Barbeau,* Clinical Research Institute, 110 Pine Avenue West, Montreal, Quebec, Canada, H2W 1R7.

Journal of Neural Transmission, Suppl. 16, 195—198 (1980)

Is the Neurosurgical Treatment
of Parkinson's Disease Still Indicated?

J. Siegfried

Department of Neurosurgery, University of Zürich, Zürich, Switzerland

With 1 Figure

Summary

Long-term results of the medical treatment of Parkinson's disease are somewhat disappointing despite an increased longevity and a more prolonged functional ability. The appearance of iatrogenic side-effects lead some authors to withhold levodopa until severity of symptoms really warrants its use. In this context the place of neurosurgery is re-evaluated. With specific indications a correctly performed stereotactic operation is still the best therapy available capable of suppressing tremor, iatrogenic hyperkinesias and rigidity and must be considered when these symptoms incapacitate the functional and social life of the patient.

Several surgical procedures were proposed for treatment of the tremor and rigidity of Parkinson's disease before the introduction of stereotactic techniques. All of these operations, although occasionally effective, caused side effects. Most prominent of these was marked weakness of the involved limb. The development of human stereotaxy in 1947 by *Spiegel et al.* opened a fascinating approach to the treatment and the physiological understanding of Parkinson's disease. Several stereotactic frames were built and various lesion techniques perfected (mechanical, chemical and physiological). This method of treatment became popular in the late 1950's, when it was proved in 1955 that a stereotactic localized destruction of the ventrolateral part of the thalamus suppressed tremor and rigidity on the opposite side in a very high percentage of cases and without neurological deficit for the whole life of patient. Subsequent to the advent of levodopa therapy, surgical treatment of Parkinson's disease has been almost discontinued. For example, prior to the development of L-dopa therapy approximately 700 operations were carried out by *Cooper* each year for the relief of Parkinsonian tremor and rigidity; since the advent of L-dopa the average annual number of cases of surgical intervention in parkinsonism has been 25 [1]. We have made similar observations (Fig. 1). After the introduction of stereotactic techniques in our department in 1958, the number of cases with Parkinsonian symptoms operated on reached a high peak in 1961, then decreased and stayed more or less constant until 1968, when we started to treat patients with L-dopa and a decarboxylase inhibitor. The number of operations performed decreased immediately. After the introduction in Switzerland of Larodopa® in 1970 and of Madopar® in 1973 the number of surgical interventions decreased even more until 1975, with the lowest peak about 10 times less than in 1963. Since 1975 neurosurgical treatment of tremor has been regularly increasing again with almost as many stereotactic operations today as before the commercial introduction of levodopa.

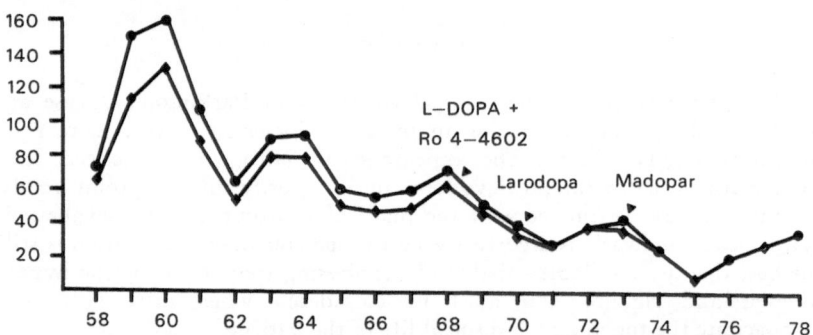

Fig. 1. Number of stereotactic operations (top line) and of patients operated on (bottom line) for Parkinson's disease in Zürich from 1958 to 1978. (Since a few years, almost no patients are operated on both sides)

This new interest in the neurosurgical treatment of Parkinson's disease can be explained by the following facts:

1. Increasing observations of cases with persistent tremor and rigidity after an extensive trial of properly supervised drug therapy.

2. More use of lower doses of levodopa to reduce the later on-off phenomenon with all their aspects and consequently less favorable effects on tremor and rigidity.

3. The indication for iatrogenic dyskinesias, when the involuntary movements to levodopa are marked on one side of the body with otherwise a satisfactory functional result. We first observed that patients, who have received unilateral stereotactic thalamic surgery

[6, 7] for the relief of tremor and rigidity before institution of L-dopa therapy rarely, if ever, develop involuntary movements as a result of L-dopa therapy. This observation was subsequently confirmed many times [1, 2, 4, 7].

4. The institution of operative procedures as first therapeutic approach, when tremor is almost the only symptom. Although it is generally stated that medicinal therapy should be given an adequate trial before surgical intervention is advised, such a sequence may be changed is such cases. Since the optimal therapeutic benefits of levodopa and of dopamine agonists occur during the first years of use and their early effectiveness is replaced by oscillations in performance and the appearance of new symptoms such as hyperkinesias and psychical alterations, it was proposed by *Rinne,* among others, not to begin the treatment in patients with mild symptoms but to withhold levodopa until severity of symptoms really warrants its use [3]. Drug therapy for Parkinson's disease has many drawbacks: it is a tedious and troublesome form of treatment which usually must be continued for an indefinite period; it can have unpleasant side effects and it is a form of control, not a cure. Stereotactic destruction of a small part of the ventrolateral thalamus or of the zona incerta controls the tremor quicker and better for the whole life time than drug therapy does.

Measuring the efficacy of surgical treatment of Parkinson's disease is much less complicated than measuring the efficacy and toxicity of an antiparkinson drug. Tremor and rigidity disappear like a blow and success is long-lasting. A correctly performed stereotactic operation is still the only therapy available capable of suppressing tremor and rigidity permanently on the operated side in about 85 % of cases [1, 5].

The indications for neurosurgical treatment of Parkinson's disease are the following:
1. Abnormal movements whose intensity justifies operative treatment.
2. a) Lack of efficiency of all known conservative procedures;
   b) As first treatment when tremor is almost the only symptom.
3. There are no contraindications such as
   organic brain syndrome
   hydrocephalus
   hypertension
   diabetes
   previous stereotactic operation on one side.

These indications must be considered when not only tremor, but also rigidity and iatrogenic dyskinesias incapacitate the functional and social life of the patient.

References

[1] *Cooper, I. S.:* Neurosurgical treatment of the dyskinesias. Clin. Neurosurg. *24*, 367—390 (1977).

[2] *Matsumoto, K., Asano, T., Bara, T., Miyamoto, T., Ohmoto, T.:* Long-term follow-up results of bilateral thalamotomy for parkinsonism. Appl. Neurophysiol. *39*, 257—260 (1976/77).

[3] *Rinne, U. K.:* Recent advances in research on parkinsonism. Acta neurol. Scand. *57*, Suppl. 67, 77—113 (1978).

[4] *Selby, G.:* The influence of previous stereotactic thalamotomy on L-dopa therapy in Parkinson's disease. Proc. Aust. Assoc. Neurol. *13*, 55—60 (1976).

[5] *Siegfried, J.:* Die Parkinsonsche Krankheit und ihre Behandlung, pp. 262. Wien: Springer. 1968.

[6] *Siegfried, J.:* Deux ans d'expérience avec la L-Dopa associée à un inhibiteur de la décarboxylase. Rev. Neurol. *122*, 243—248 (1970).

[7] *Siegfried, J.:* The place of L-Dopa in the treatment of Parkinson's disease. Progr. Neurol. Surg. *5*, 387—405 (1973).

[8] *Siegfried, J., Klaiber, R., Ziegler, W. H.:* Induced abnormal movements with L-dopa and Ro 4-4602. In: L-DOPA and Parkinsonism (*Barbeau, A., McDowell, F. H.*, eds.), pp. 114—118. Philadelphia: F. A. Davis. 1970.

Authors' address: Prof. Dr. *J. Siegfried*, Neurosurgical Clinic, University of Zürich School of Medicine, Raemistrasse 100, CH-8091 Zürich, Switzerland.

Journal of Neural Transmission, Suppl. 16, 199—210 (1980)
© by Springer-Verlag 1980

Benign and Malignant Types of Parkinson's Disease: Clinical and Patho-Physiological Characterization

W. Danielczyk, P. Riederer, and D. Seemann

Department of Neurology, Lainz Geriatric Hospital, and Neurochemistry Group, Ludwig Boltzmann-Institute of Clinical Neurobiology, Lainz-Hospital, Wien, Austria

With 1 Figure

Summary

Parkinson's disease (P.D.) is characterized by two different types, a benign form found in 85 % of patients and a malignant type in 15 %. Computer tomography shows malignant patients, in the end stage of the disease process, to exhibit hydrocephalus internus *and* externus. Such patients exhibit early EEG-deterioration and pharmacotoxic psychosis.

The application of neuroleptics to patients with P.D. is associated with an increase in the urinary excretion of acidic metabolites especially of 5-hydroxyindoleacetic acid. It is suggested, that this treatment might also be a useful therapeutic approach to optimizing the residual neuronal function in Parkinson's disease.

Key words: Parkinson's disease, computer tomography, neuroleptics, EEG.

Introduction

There is no doubt that the atrophy of the melanin-containing cells of the substantia nigra plays a significant role in the aetiology of Parkinson's disease (P.D.). This degeneration affects the dopaminergic neurons of the striatum which exhibit a substantial reduction of the rate-limiting enzyme in catecholamine synthesis, tyrosine hydroxylase (*Lloyd* and *Hornykiewicz*, 1975; *Nagatsu et al.*, 1977; *Riederer et al.*, 1978) and its pteridin-cofactor BH_4 (*Levine et al.*, 1979) and disturbs important functions of neurotransmission in dopamine neurons including storage capacity and presynaptic neuronal activity; yet a loss of activity in the dopamine-metabolizing enzyme monoamine oxidase has not been observed (*Bernheimer et al.*, 1962).

Animal models to simulate P.D. lead to the hypothesis that a degeneration of presynaptic dopaminergic nerve terminals causes supersensitivity of postsynaptic dopamine neurons, thus to some extent compensating for the loss of functional neural capacity (*Unger-stedt*, 1970). In fact a compensatory neuronal overactivity has been found in P.D. There is an increased turnover of dopamine (*Bern-heimer et al.*, 1973) and, in some brain areas, of noradrenaline (*Riederer et al.*, 1977), results consistent with the predominant nerve cell loss of the substantia nigra and locus coeruleus in P.D. (for review *Bernheimer et al.*, 1973). Since the early days of replacing the deficiency of dopamine by L-DOPA (a precursor amino-acid of the catecholamines), this treatment, with or without the combination of peripherally acting decarboxylase inhibitors, has been the basic therapy for P.D. (*Birkmayer* and *Hornykiewicz*, 1961; *Barbeau et al.*, 1961; *Birkmayer* and *Mentasti*, 1967). However this has been supplemented by anticholinergics, the MAO-inhibitors (—)Deprenyl (*Birk-mayer et al.*, 1975 a) and Parnate®, dopaminergic agonists like alpha-ergobromocriptine (*Calne et al.*, 1974) and lisuride (*Parkes*, 1979; *Calne*, 1979) and amantadine (*Schwab et al.*, 1969), such dopamin-ergic stimulants being specially applicable in the "decompensated phase" of P.D. (*Yahr*, 1979).

Through such combined treatment the symptoms exhibited by patients can be substantially diminished. Duration and progression of the disease, however, cannot be influenced in a decisive manner (*Birkmayer et al.*, 1974 a). As the disease progresses and patients disabilities change individually, drug treatment can be difficult (*Birkmayer* and *Riederer*, 1980). Moreover about 10—15 % of patients with P.D. are resistant to such therapy, this being observed soon after the diagnosis of the disease ("malignant types") (*Birkmayer et al.*, 1974 a), as well as in the end stage of the disease, when "benign types" (duration of the disease between 10 and 15 years), become akinetic and rigid non-responders. Therefore, it is of interest to differentiate these benign and malignant types of P.D. and this should be possible in a department for chronical neurological diseases where patients are hospitalized over many years.

Materials and Methods

At the end of 1979 58 patients with Parkinson's disease were hospitalized in our department.

For clinical reasons drug treatment was continued during the study, except for L-DOPA, or combined DOPA-treatment, which was witheld for 2 days before collection of blood and urine. Clinical criteria were assessed using the Webster rating scale and a special rating scale for determining motor behaviour of the patients (*Birkmayer* and *Neumayer, 1972*).

Computed tomography (C.T.) and EEG were performed to assess brain anatomy and function in 48 parkinsonian patients. 39 suffered from idiopathic parkinsonism, 1 from postencephalitic and 8 had a senile type with arteriosclerotic manifestation.

Five patients with benign and 5 patients with malignant type of idiopathic P.D. have been selected in a random fashion. The leading criterion for selection was the duration of drug response to combined L-DOPA preparations or other types of usual antiparkinson therapies, as mentioned above.

Patients who develop high disability (70 or more, according to *Birkmayer et al.*, 1974 a) within the first 5 years and did not respond to any drug treatment, were characterized as malignant, whereas patients with a disease duration of more than 10 years and good response to drug treatment were defined as having benign type of P.D.

Serum dopamine and noradrenaline have been determined in all 10 patients by using HPLC-electrochemical detection as described by *Reynolds et al.* (in preparation).

Acidic metabolites, homovanillic acid, vanilmandelic acid and 5-hydroxyindoleacetic acid have been measured by HPLC with UV-detection. In brief, the acidified urine was extracted twice with diethyl ether, the combined fractions taken to dryness, dissolved into 0.2 M acetic acid and 20 μl injected. The eluting medium was 0.2 M acetic acid (*Riederer et al.*, in preparation).

Results

After dividing the patients into two groups as described above, the following results were obtained:

The mean age of the patients at the time of the rating was, for benign cases 68 ± 2.2 years and for the malignant patients 73.8 ± 2.3 years, the mean age at the onset of the disease was 53.4 ± 3.4 (benign) and 72.2 ± 2.3 (malignant), respectively.

The duration of the disease at the time of the rating was 14.6 ± 3 years for benign and 3.6 ± 0.4 years for malignant cases. The disability at the time of the rating was 48 ± 10, for benign and 70 ± 5.4 for malignant cases.

C.T.'s showed hydrocephalus internus *and* externus for malignant patients, whereas 4 out of 5 patients with benign P.D had only hydrocephalus internus (Fig. 1 a and b).

In benign cases 3 had the EEG-alpha-reaction, whereas in malignant cases the alpha-reaction could not be seen in 4 out of

Table 1. *Clinical and pathophysiological characterization of benign and malignant types of Parkinson's disease*

	Patients									
	1	2	3	4	5	6	7	8	9	10
Year of birth	1912	1906	1901	1902	1919	1912	1909	1903	1898	1909
Sex	F	F	F	M	F	F	F	F	F	F
Onset of P.D.-year	1976	1968	1976	1975	1960	1965	1964	1974	1976	1965
Symptomatic	akin.	hyperkin.	akin.	akin.	akin.	akin.	akin.	akin.	akin.	akin.
Benign or malignant	—	+	—	—	+	+	+	—	—	+
Disability*	50	80	80	70	20	50	30	70	80	60
C.T.	HI+E	HI+E	HI+E	HI+E	HI	HI	NP	HI+E	HI+E	NP
EEG	+++	+++	+++	++	++	++	++	+++	+	++
Alpha-reaction	—	—	—	—	—	—	+	—	+	+
Pharmacotoxic psychosis	+	+	+	+	+++	+++	—	+	—	—
L-DOPA	—	+++	—	—	+	+++	—	—	—	—
Combined L-DOPA**	—	+++	+++	+	—	+++	++	—	—	+
Amantadine	+	+	—	—	+	+	—	+	—	+
Antidholinergics	—	—	—	—	—	—	—	—	+	+
α-ergobromocriptine	—	+++	—	—	—	+	—	—	—	—
MAO-inhibitors***	—	+++	—	—	++	—	+	—	—	+
Antidepressants	—	+++	+	+	—	+	—	—	—	—
Neuroleptics	—	+	—	—	—	—	—	+	—	—

Pharmacotoxic psychosis: — not observed, + sensitive to. Akin. = akinetic type of P.D. Hyperkin. = hyperkinetic type of P.D. P.D. = Parkinson's disease. C.T. = computed tomography. Medication according to usual clinical practice: benign: +, malignant: —. EEG: minor irregular slow activity: +, moderate irregular slow activity: ++, major irregular slow activity: +++. Psych. = pharmacotoxic psychosis. Alpha-reaction: positiv: +, negativ: —. HI+E = hydrocephalus internus + externus. NP = not present. Drug treatment: present +, absent —.
* According to *Birkmayer* and *Neumayer* (1972). ** Madopar®. *** (—)Deprenyl, Parnate.

5 patients. In benign cases the psychotic phases were observed only in 2 patients, whereas in malignant cases 4 out of the 5 patients suffered from pharmacotoxic psychosis. The patient who did not show this side effect, was treated with neither DOPA-preparations nor amantadine.

Biochemical determinations of dopamine and noradrenaline in plasma and their metabolites in urine did not show substantial differences between benign and malignant types of P.D. (results not shown), however the limited number of patients in both groups does not allow any conclusive statement regarding catecholamine metabolism in these patients.

Table 2 shows that drug treatment has a substantial influence on the concentration of acidic metabolites. The lowest concentration of metabolites was observed in patients treated with amantadine and anticholinergics, whereas the highest excretion was observable in patients who were on additional neuroleptic treatment. No differences however can be shown between benign and malignant types of P.D.

Table 2. *Acid amine metabolites during neuroleptic drug treatment*

		Parkinson's disease	
	Controls (9)	Non-clopenthixol (5)	Clopenthixol (5)
Homovanillic acid	4.5 ± 1.0	3.98 ± 1.46	6.44 ± 2.03
Vanilmandelic acid	10.5 ± 4.7	16.57 ± 5.30	23.5 ± 5.70
5-hydroxyindole- acetic acid	2.3 ± 0.3	0.72 ± 0.20	13.15 ± 4.76*

Number of patients in parenthesis. Means ± s.e.m.; mg/24 hours.

At the time of urine collection all parkinsonian patients were withdrawn from any L-DOPA medication, but were on a basic antiparkinson therapy with amantadine and anticholinergics. Clopenthixol medication was 15 to 30 mg/day.

* $p < 0.01$ versus controls and patients not treated with clopenthixol.

Discussion

Malignant types of P.D. can be characterized preferentially by clinical ratings, although a number of tests, like C.T., EEG and biochemical data may be of additional help. In an earlier study *Birkmayer et al.* (1979) have shown that malignant types of P.D. do not exist preferentially in older patients. Therefore a distinction into

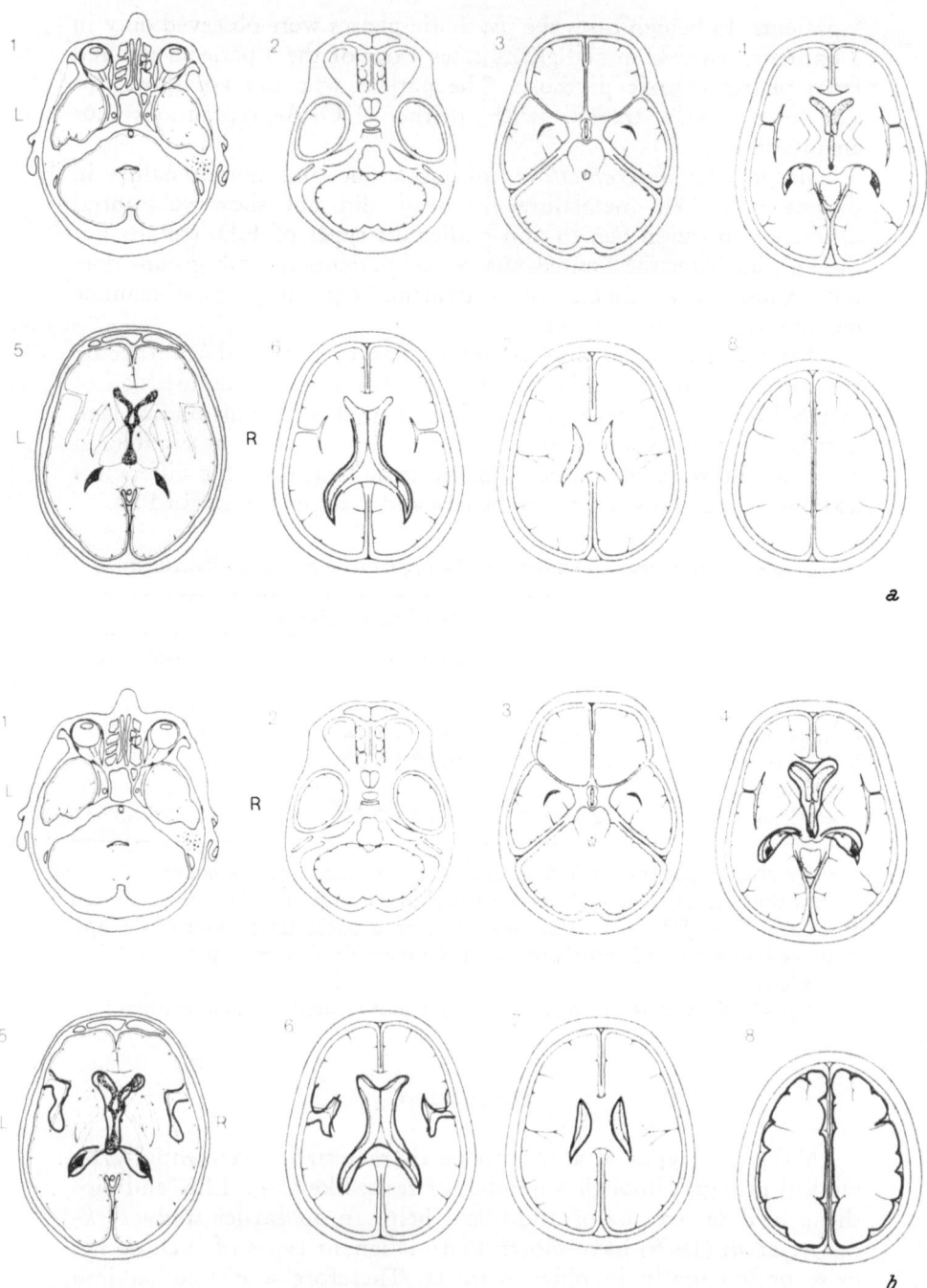

benign and malignant types of P.D. is justified. However, his and our data clearly demonstrate that at higher age the possibility for a malignant type of P.D. is significantly higher than for young patients.

This finding is of special interest and demonstrates that the normal "aging" of dopamine neurons seems to play an important role in P.D. It has been shown by *Bertler* (1961), *Carlsson* and *Winblad* (1976), *Riederer* and *Wuketich* (1976), that dopamine concentrations in human brain decrease with age. Moreover, dynamic measurement demonstrated not only a nonlinear decrease of dopamine (*Riederer* and *Wuketich*, 1976), but also for tyrosine hydroxylase (*McGeer et al.*, 1973), the rate limiting enzyme in catecholamine synthesis and in the cofactor BH_4 (*Levine et al.*, 1979).

Thus we feel, it is reasonable to suggest that the disability of contracting malignant P.D. is increased with age. There is recent evidence that in P.D. not only a degeneration of presynaptic dopaminergic nerve terminals occurs, but that also postsynaptic dopamine receptors lose sensitivity (*Reisine et al.*, 1977; *Riederer et al.*, 1978; *Shibuya*, 1979; *Rinne et al.*, 1979; *Spokes*, 1979; *Riederer et al.*, 1980). It could be, however, that postsynaptic receptors or neurons degenerate much faster in malignant cases than in benign P.D. Support for this hypothesis stems from one case with clinical symptoms of P.D. who did not respond to any drug treatment. Dopamine receptor binding in post-mortem brain tissue was by far lower than usually observed (*Reynolds et al.*, 1980). Histological examination (*Jellinger et al.*, 1980) showed that this patient suffered from supranuclear palsy. Therefore, it cannot be excluded that some other diseases with similar clinical characteristics are combined with P.D. and that these secondary diseases facilitate the malignant response to any drug treatment (*Lieberman et al.*, 1979). It is a common clinical experience that malignant types of P.D. in long-term hospitalization do not show significant improvement of motor performance when treated with dopamine stimulants. They do, however, develop pharmacotoxic psychoses (*Danielczyk*, 1979).

EEG-studies show diminished or absent alpha-reaction in malignant cases and this might be correlated with the C.T. findings showing hydrocephalus internus *and* externus to a high degree.

Fig. 1. *a* Patient A.L., female 70 years. Diagnosis: Parkinson's disease (benign form). Normal C.T. for age. Calcification of the pineal body and chorioid plexus. *b* Patient W.L., female 76 years. Diagnosis: Parkinson's disease (malignant form). Predominant cortical atrophy, particularly in the sulci and interhemispheral space (respectively 8 and 9 mm). Widening of the ventricular system; cellae mediae index 3.5

The development of cortical as well as ventricular atrophies seems to be more significant in geriatric long-term hospitalized patients (*Reisner et al.*, 1979). *Schwab et al.* (1959) tried to correlate ventricular atrophies with akinesia and *Selby* (1968) found a high correlation between cortical atrophy and rigidity using pneumoencephalographic measurement. Recently, *Fischer et al.* (1976), *Becker et al.* (1979) and *Schneider et al.* (1979), showed that cortical atrophy might have more importance than ventricular atrophy in P.D.

50 to 60 % of P.D.-patients suffer from dementia. It has been shown, by histological examination, that combined P.D.-dementia-patients show changes in the frontal cortex, hippocampus, nucleus amygdala and thalamus, as well in the substantia nigra, locus coeruleus, reticular substance, tegmentum and vagal nucleus (*Black-wood*, 1979). The extranigral lesions might also contribute to the sensitivity of P.D.-patients to pharmacotoxic psychosis (*Birkmayer et al.*, 1974, 1975). In contrast to malignant types of P.D., the benign types respond to dopamine stimulants in the long-term treatment and to amantadine infusions in the beginning of akinetic crises (*Danielczyk*, 1973). The end stage of benign P.D., however, is a developing akinetic crisis which does not respond to any drug treatment (80 % in our material). The time course of P.D. can, however be benign (85 %) or malignant (15 %).

Measurements of catecholamines and their metabolites in peripheral fluids reflect, on the whole, peripheral and not central changes. As such parameters seem here to change with drug treatment, this findings suggest a possible involvement of medication on the peripheral neuronal tissue. It is therefore, of interest to note that neuroleptic drug treatment increases the concentration of transmitter metabolites in the urines of our patients. Recently, post-mortem studies have shown that neuroleptic drug treatment increases the number of D_2-receptors in the striatum of parkinsonian patients (*Rinne et al.*, 1979).

Neuroleptic and antiparkinson therapy might contribute to a prolonged stimulation of motor-performance on the basis that the normally decreased receptor numbers (*Reisine et al.*, 1977), can be overcome by neuroleptic treatment. The application of neuroleptics with a resultant increased receptor number may be a useful therapeutic approach to optimizing the residual dopaminergic function in P.D. However, the end stage of P.D. as well as the malignant types of P.D. are characterized by akinetic crises and pharmacotoxic psychosis (*Danielczyk*, 1980). Therefore the treatment of such patients with drugs stimulating dopamine neurons and, at the same time, with low dosage of neuroleptics like clopenthixol (15—30 mg a day) which block postsynaptic receptors, is a strategy between "Scylla and Charybdis", but may relieve the symptoms and prolong life for as long as possible.

Acknowledgements

We are grateful to Prof. Dr. K. Fochem for the C.T.'s, to Dr. G. Reynolds for biochemical assays and for his help during the preparation of the manuscript and to G. Stift for secretarial work.

References

Barbeau, A., Murphy, G. F., Sourkes, T. L.: Excretion of dopamine in diseases of basal ganglia. Science *133,* 1706—1707 (1961).

Becker, H., Schneider, E., Hacker, H., Fischer, P. A.: Cerebral atrophy in Parkinson's disease—represented in CT. Arch. Psychiatr. Nervenkr. *227,* 81—88 (1979).

Bernheimer, H., Birkmayer, W., Hornykiewicz, O.: Verhalten der Monoaminoxydase im Gehirn des Menschen nach Therapie mit Monoaminoxydase-Hemmern. Wien. klin. Wschr. *74,* 558—559 (1962).

Bernheimer, H., Birkmayer, W., Hornykiewicz, O., Jellinger, K., Seitelberger, F.: Brain dopamine and the syndromes of Parkinson and Huntington. J. neurol. Sci. *20,* 415—455 (1973).

Bertler, A.: Occurrence and localization of catecholamines in the human brain. Acta physiol. Scand. *51,* 97—107 (1961).

Birkmayer, W., Hornykiewicz, O.: Der L-Dioxyphenylalanin (L-DOPA)-Effekt bei der Parkinson-Akinese. Wien. klin. Wschr. *73,* 787—788 (1961).

Birkmayer, W., Mentasti, M.: Weitere experimentelle Untersuchungen über den Catecholaminstoffwechsel bei extrapyramidalen Erkrankungen. Arch. Psychiatr. Nervenkr. *210,* 29—35 (1967).

Birkmayer, W., Neumayer, E.: Die moderne medikamentöse Behandlung des Parkinsonismus. Z. Neurol. *202,* 257—280 (1972).

Birkmayer, W., Danielczyk, W., Neumayer, E., Riederer, P.: Nucleus ruber and L-DOPA-psychosis—biochemical post-mortem findings. J. Neural Transm. *35,* 93—116 (1974).

Birkmayer, W., Neumayer, E., Ambrozi, L., Riederer, P.: Longevity in Parkinson's disease treated with L-DOPA. Clin. Neurol. Neurosurg. *1,* 15—19 (1974 a).

Birkmayer, W., Riederer, P.: Responsibility of extrastriatal areas for the appearance of psychotic symptoms. J. Neural Transm. *37,* 175—182 (1975).

Birkmayer, W., Riederer, P., Youdim, M. B. H., Linauer, W.: Potentiation of the anti-akinetic effect after L-DOPA treatment by an inhibitor of MAO-B, Deprenyl. J. Neural Transm. *36,* 303—323 (1975).

Birkmayer, W., Riederer, P., Rausch, W. D.: Neuropharmacological principles and problems of combined treatment in Parkinson's disease. In: Adv. Neurol., Vol. 24 (*Poirier, L. J., Sourkes, T. L., Bedard, P. J.*, eds.), pp. 499—510. New York: Raven Press. 1979.

Birkmayer, W., Riederer, P.: Die Parkinson-Krankheit. Wien: Springer. 1980 (in preparation).

Blackwood, W.: Morbid anatomy. Int. Symp. on Progress in Parkinson's disease research. London, 12—14 December 1979, Pitman Medical (in press).

Calne, D. B., Teychenne, P. F., Claveria, L. E., Eastman, R., Greenacre, J. K., Petrie, A.: Bromocriptine in Parkinsonism. Brit. Med. J. *4*, 442—444 (1974).

Calne, D. B.: Bromocriptine and other dopaminergic ergot derivatives. Int. Symp. on progress in Parkinson's disease research. London, 12—14 December 1979, Pitman Medical (in press).

Carlsson, A., Winblad, B.: Influence of age and time interval between death and autopsy on dopamine and 3-methoxytyramine levels in human basal ganglia. J. Neural Transm. *38*, 271—276 (1976).

Danielczyk, W.: Akute pharmakotoxische Psychosen bei chronischen cerebralen Erkrankungen. Wien. med. Wschr. *129*, Suppl. 55 (1979).

Danielczyk, W.: Die Behandlung von akinetischen Krisen. Med. Welt *24* (N.F.), 1278—1282 (1973).

Danielczyk, W.: Krisen im Verlauf des Morbus Parkinson. Wien. med. Wschr. 1980 (in press).

Fischer, P. A., Jacobi, P., Schneider, E., Becker, H.: Correlation between clinical and CT-findings in Parkinson's syndrome. In: Cranial Computerized Tomography (*Lanksch, N., Kazner, E.*, eds.), pp. 246—248. Berlin-Heidelberg-New York: Springer. 1976.

Jellinger, K., Riederer, P., Tomonaga, M.: Progressive supranuclear palsy: Clinico-pathological and biochemical studies. J. Neural Transm., Suppl. *16*, 111—128 (1980).

Levine, R. A., Williams, A. C., Robinson, D. S., Calne, D. B., Lovenberg, W.: Analysis of hydroxylase cofactor activity in the cerebrospinal fluid of patients with Parkinson's disease. In: Adv. Neurol., Vol. 24 (*Poirier, L. J., Sourkes, T. L., Bedard, P. J.*, eds.), pp. 203—207. New York: Raven Press. 1979.

Lieberman, A., Dziatolowski, M., Kupersmith, M., Serby, M., Goodgold, A., Korein, J., Goldstein, M.: Dementia in Parkinson's disease. Ann. Neurol. *6*, 355—359 (1979).

Lloyd, K. G., Davidson, L., Hornykiewicz, O.: The neurochemistry of Parkinson's disease: Effect of L-DOPA therapy. J. Pharmacol. Exp. Ther. *195*, 453—464 (1975).

McGeer, E. G., McGeer, P. L.: Some characteristics of brain tyrosine hydroxylase. In: New Concepts in Neurotransmitter Regulation (*Mandell, A. J.*, ed.), pp. 53—68. Plenum Press. 1973.

Nagatsu, T., Numata, Y., Ikuta, K., Sano, M., Nagatsu, I., Kondo, Y., Inagaki, S., Ilzuka, R., Hori, A., Narabayashi, H.: Phenylethanolamine-N-Methyltransferase and other enzymes of catecholamine metabolism in human brain. Clin. chim. Acta *75,* 221—232 (1977).

Parkes, J.: Lisuride and bromocriptine. Int. Symp. on Progress in Parkinson's disease research. London, 12—14 December 1979, Pitman Medical (in press).

Reisine, T. D., Fields, J. Z., Stern, L. Z., Johnson, P. C., Bird, E. D., Yamamura, H. I.: Alterations in dopaminergic receptors in Huntington's disease. Life Sciences *21,* 1123—1128 (1977).

Reisner, Th., Brunner, G., Schnaberth, G.: Computertomographische Erfassung der malignen Verlaufsform des Parkinson-Syndroms. Kongressband, deutsch-österreichische Neurologentagung, Oktober 1979, Wien (in press).

Reynolds, G. P., Riederer, P., Owen, F., Cross, A. J., Crow, T.: In preparation (1980).

Riederer, P., Wuketich, St.: Time course of nigrostriatal degeneration in Parkinson's disease. J. Neural Transm. *38,* 277—301 (1976).

Riederer, P., Birkmayer, W., Seemann, D., Wuketich, St.: Brain noradrenaline and 3-methoxy-4-hydroxyphenylglycol in Parkinson's syndrome. J. Neural Transm. *41,* 241—251 (1977).

Riederer, P., Rausch, W. D., Birkmayer, W., Jellinger, K., Danielczyk, W.: Dopamine-sensitive adenylate cyclase activity in the caudate nucleus and adrenal medulla in Parkinson's disease and in liver cirrhosis. J. Neural Transm., Suppl. *14,* 153—161 (1978).

Riederer, P., Rausch, W. D., Birkmayer, W., Jellinger, K., Seemann, D.: CNS modulation of adrenal tyrosine hydroxylase in Parkinson's disease and metabolic encephalopathies. J. Neural Transm., Suppl. *14,* 121—131 (1978).

Riederer, P., Reynolds, G. P., Birkmayer, W.: Neurochemical correlates of symptomatology and drug induced side effects in Parkinson's disease. In: Progress in Parkinson's Disease Research. Pitman Medical (1980, in press).

Rinne, U. K., Sonninen, V., Laaksonen, H.: Responses of brain neurochemistry to levodopa treatment in Parkinson's disease. In: Adv. Neurol., Vol. 24 *(Poirier, L. J., Sourkes, T. L., Bedard, P. J.,* eds.), pp. 259—274. New York: Raven Press. 1979.

Schneider, E., Becker, H., Fischer, P. A., Grau, H., Jakobi, P., Brinkmann, R.: The course of brain atrophy in Parkinson's disease. Arch. Psychiat. Nervenkr. *227,* 89—95 (1979).

Schwab, R. S., England, A. C., Peterson, E.: Akinesia in Parkinson's disease. Neurology (Minneap.) *9,* 65—72 (1959).

Schwab, R. S., Poshanzer, D. C.: Amantadine in the treatment of Parkinson's disease. J. Amer. Med. Ass. *208,* 1168 (1969).

Shibuya, M.: Dopamine-sensitive adenylate cyclase activity in the striatum in Parkinson's disease. J. Neural Transm. *44,* 287—295 (1979), presented in the 4th int. catecholamine symp., 17—22 September 1978, Asimolar, U.S.A.

Spokes, E. G. S.: Dopamine and dopamine receptor binding. Int. Symp. on Progress in Parkinson's disease research, London, 12—14 December 1979, Pitman Medical (in press).

Selby, G.: Cerebral atrophy in Parkinsonism. J. Neurol. Sci. *6*, 517—559 (1968).

Ungerstedt, U., Arbuthnott, G. W.: Quantitative recording of rotional behaviour in rats after 6-OH dopamine lesions of the nigrostriatal dopamine system. Brain Res. *24*, 485—493 (1970).

Winkler, M. H., Berl, S., Whetsell, W. O., Yahr, M. D.: Spiroperidol binding in the human caudate nucleus. J. Neural Transm., Suppl. *16*, 45—51 (1980).

Yahr, M. D.: Initiation of treatment. Int. Symp. on Progress in Parkinson's disease research, London, 12—14 December 1979. London: Pitman Medical (in press).

Authors' address: Doz. Dr. *W. Danielczyk*, Neurological Department, Lainz Geriatric Hospital, Versorgungsheimplatz 1, A-1130 Wien, Austria.

Journal of Neural Transmission, Suppl. 16, 211—215 (1980)

Theoretical and Clinical Aspects of the Tourette Syndrome (Chronic Multiple Tic)

R. Fog and H. Pakkenberg

St. Hans Hospital, Department E, Roskilde, and Department of Neurology, Hvidovre Hospital, Denmark

Summary

In three schizophrenic patients long-term neuroleptic treatment induced Tourette-like symptoms. There seems to be a partial overlap in the pathogenesis of Tourette syndrome and tardive dyskinesia.

In five Tourette patients treatment with pimozide was very effective inducing only few side-effects. Long-term neuroleptic treatment may, however, aggravate the symptoms in the long run.

A combination treatment with tetrabenazine and pimozide is suggested.

Introduction

The Tourette syndrome bridges the gap between neurology and psychiatry. The syndrome is characterized by childhood onset of chronic motor tics and involuntary vocalizations—in many cases of obscene words (coprolalia). Both types of symptoms are in about 80 % of the cases successfully treated with haloperidol (*Brunn et al.*, 1976). Other antidopaminergic drugs are also effective and therefore, a "dopamine hypothesis" has been developed for the Tourette syndrome (*Snyder et al.*, 1970; *Butler et al.*, 1979).

The lifelong nature of the disorder may necessitate prolonged treatment which increases the risk for onset of tardive dyskinesia (*Gerlach*, 1979). There seems to be a partial overlap between tardive dyskinesia and Tourette syndrome: In this paper we will describe some cases of schizophrenic patients who have developed Tourette-like symptoms after treatment for years with antidopaminergic drugs.

In the treatment of Tourette patients haloperidol is the most widely used antidopaminergic drug. Haloperidol has, however, some sedative effects and may also give rise to Parkinsonian side-effects. In an open study we treated patients with pimozide, which is a strong antidopaminergic agent related to haloperidol, but with fewer side-effects. The results were encouraging and are also reported in this paper.

Material

1. Schizophrenic Patients with Neuroleptic Induced Tourette-Like Symptoms

Case 1 (J.L.): Schizophrenic symptoms (simple form) since age of 17, now 20 years old. For two years treated with haloperidol 4—10 mg daily. In relation to discontinuation of haloperidol development of tics of head and body accompanied by grunting. The symptoms diminished, when haloperidol was reinstituted.

Case 2 (A.B.): Schizophrenic symptoms (paranoid form) since age of 40, now 56 years old. Since age of 40 treated with various neuroleptic drugs, mostly phenothiazines and haloperidol. From age of 54 sudden short spells of arm movements, words, and echolalia but also of slamming doors and shouting. The symptoms diminished on treatment with pimozide 6 mg daily (which also controls the schizophrenic symptoms). Now treated for 3 months.

Case 3 (E.S.): Schizophrenic symptoms (paranoid form) since age of 41, now 53 years old. Since age of 42 treated with various neuroleptic drugs, mostly phenothiazines. Some tendency of echopraxia (involuntary imitation of the movements of others) already in childhood, but from age of 50 aggravation with many spells of echopraxia, echolalia and howling. Has never had tics, but during the last few years oral dyskinesias. Symptoms have nearly disappeared on treatment with pimozide 6 mg daily, now for 5 months.

2. Tourette Patients Treated with Pimozide

Case 1 (H. J.): Since age of 16 periods of tics of head, stammering, grunting, coughing and echopraxia and echolalia. Now 26 years old. Perphenazine treatment was without effect. For two years treated successfully with pimozide 2 mg daily. Complained of tiredness. No aggravation for 1 1/2 years after discontinuation of pimozide.

Case 2 (M.S.): Since age of 7 (now 15) dyskinesia-like tics of face (mouth, tongue, eyes) and sounds. Very successfully treated for two months with pimozide 2 mg daily. Complained of tiredness. Only a few tics reappeared after discontinuation of pimozide (observation period one year).

Case 3 (A.J.): Since age of 9 (now 11) multiple tics and sounds. Treated with haloperidol but developed Parkinsonian side-effects. For one year treated successfully with pimozide 0.5—1.5 mg daily. Nearly all symptoms have disappeared.

Case 4 (B.S.): Since age of 5 (now 15) in relation to rheumatic fever multiple tics, hick-ups, sounds and later coprolalia. Some aggressive tendencies which led to psychiatric hospitalization. Treated with haloperidol but developed allergy. Pimozide treatment 8 mg daily for 4 months have controlled all symptoms.

Case 5 (D.S.): Since age of 4 (now 19) spells of screaming restlessness and tics. No symptoms from age 14—17. Now for 1 1/2 years treated with pimozide 2 mg daily. Sounds have disappeared but still some tics.

Results

In the three schizophrenic patients long-term neuroleptic treatment seems to have induced Tourette-like symptoms. Case 3 has, however, never had any tics but showed oral dyskinesia. All patients benefited by treatment with pimozide.

In the five Tourette patients treated with pimozide nearly all symptoms were controlled. The side-effects, especially hypokinesia, were less than with other antidopaminergic drugs even if some patients complained of tiredness.

Discussion

A hyperfunction of the dopaminergic system in the brain has been suggested in the pathogenesis of Tourette syndrome. This theory is supported by the fact that other hyperkinetic syndromes such as Huntington's chorea and tardive dyskinesia show symptoms with some resemblance to Tourette's disease. Furthermore it seems that all hyperkinesias successfully can be treated with antidopaminergic drugs (*Fog* and *Pakkenberg*, 1970; *Gerlach*, 1979).

It is often difficult to distinguish between schizophrenic stereotypies and Tourette-like symptoms. In our schizophrenic patients, however, the symptoms appeared after long-term treatment with neuroleptics accompanied by oral dyskinesia in one patient. It, therefore, seems reasonable to associate these symptoms with tardive dyskinesia.

Tardive dyskinesia has been attributed to dopaminergic supersensitivity (*Christensen*, 1979) and also to loss of cells in the basal ganglia (*Pakkenberg et al.*, 1973; *Fog* and *Pakkenberg*, 1979). Long-term neuroleptic treatment might, therefore, aggravate the symptoms in the long run (*Gerlach*, 1979).

In our patients with Tourette symptoms pimozide was able to control most symptoms inducing only few side-effects. If there is a partial overlap in the pathogenesis of Tourette syndrome and tardive dyskinesia this treatment (and any other dopamine receptor blocking treatment) may, however, aggravate the symptoms after some years (*Gibson*, 1979).

In some earlier investigations of the treatment of Huntington's chorea (*Fog* and *Pakkenberg*, 1970) and spontaneous oral dyskinesia (*Pakkenberg* and *Fog*, 1974) we have suggested a combination treatment of tetrabenazine (which inhibits the storage of dopamine in the presynaptic neuron) and pimozide (which blocks the dopamine receptor in the postsynaptic neuron). Both drugs have antidopaminergic properties, but in different ways. The clinical effect seems more lasting and the effective doses of both drugs in this combination are rather low, which also might be an advantage in long-term treatment.

References

Butler, I. J., Koslow, S. H., Seifert, W. E., jr., et al.: Biogenic amine metabolism in Tourette syndrome. Ann. Neurol. *6*, 37—39 (1979).

Brunn, R. D., Shapiro, A. K., et al.: A followup of 78 patients with Gilles de la Tourette syndrome. Am. J. Psychiatry *133*, 944—947 (1976).

Christensen, A. V., Møller, N. I.: Dopaminergic supersensitivity: Influence of dopamine agonists, cholinergics, anticholinergics and drugs used for the treatment of tardive dyskinesia. Psychopharmacology *62*, 111—116 (1979).

Fog, R., Pakkenberg, H.: Combined nitoman-pimozide treatment of Huntington's chorea and other hyperkinetic syndromes. Acta neurol. scand. *46*, 249—251 (1970).

Fog, R., Pakkenberg, H.: Combination treatment of hyperkinetic syndromes with tetrabenazine and pimozide. In: Tardive Dyskinesia (*Davis, J. M., Fann, W. E., Smith, R. C.,* eds.). New York: Spectrum Publications. 1979, in press.

Gerlach, J.: Tardive dyskinesia. Dan. Med. Bull. *26*, 209—245 (1979).

Gibson, A.: A comparison of different neuroleptic drugs and different ways of using neuroleptic drugs in the treatment of early tardive dyskinesia. In: Phenothiazines and Structurally Related Drugs. Basic and Clinical Studies (*Usdin, E., Eckert, H., Forrest, I.,* eds.). New York: Elsevier North-Holland. 1979 (in press).

Pakkenberg, H., Fog, R.: Spontaneous oral dyskinesia. Results of treatment with tetrabenazine, pimozide, or both. Arch. Neurol. *31*, 352—353 (1974).

Pakkenberg, H., Fog, R., Nilakantan, B.: The long-term effect of perphenazine enanthate on the rat brain. Some metabolic and anatomical observations. Psychopharmacologia (Berl.) *29*, 329—336 (1973).

Snyder, S. H., Taylor, K. M., Coyle, J. T., et al.: The role of brain dopamine in behavioral regulation and the actions of psychotropic drugs. Am. J. Psychiatry *127*, 199—207 (1970).

Authors' address: *H. Pakkenberg,* M.D., Laboratory of Neurology, Hvidovre Hospital, DK-2650 Hvidovre, Denmark.

Journal of Neural Transmission, Suppl. 16, 217—227 (1980)

The Neuropathology of GABA Neurons in Extrapyramidal Disorders

K. G. Lloyd

Department of Neuropharmacology, Synthélabo–L.E.R.S., Bagneux, France

Summary

Dysfunction of neurons in the extrapyramidal system (EPS) which use GABA as their neurotransmitter can be noted in both degenerative diseases of the EPS and in iatrogenic (*i.e.* drug-induced) disorders of EPS function. In Huntington's chorea there is a loss of both GABA neurons and GABA receptors in the striatum; those remaining GABA receptors likely have an altered kinetic profile, with a higher affinity for GABA than the receptors found in the non-Huntington's brain. In Parkinson's disease the lower levels of L-glutamic acid decarboxylase observed in the EPS is likely not associated with neuronal cell loss but is likely secondary to the dopamine neuron loss. These alterations in GABA neuron function and the long-term changes associated with chronic L-DOPA therapy may be related to Parkinsonian tremor. The drug-induced dyskinesias (L-DOPA, neuroleptic) appear to be associated with a relative hypo-function of EPS GABA neurons, especially in relation to DA neuron function, whereas in the case of drug-induced Parkinsonism the opposite may be the case. The function and dysfunction of GABA neurons in the EPS cannot be seen as a separate entity, but must be considered in relation to alterations in other EPS neurons, especially dopamine and acetylcholine.

A. Anatomy of GABA-Ergic Neurons in the Extrapyramidal System

The evidence for the existence of GABA-ergic neurons in the extrapyramidal system (EPS) has become very convincing during the past few years, and shows that such neurons exist as both local circuit neurons (interneurons), neurons which communicate between different

15*

nuclei of the EPS, and possibly neurons which act as efferent pathways out of the EPS (cf. *Lloyd*, 1980). GABA-ergic interneurons likely occur within the neostriatum (caudate nucleus-putamen) as in laboratory animals lesions of afferent paths to this region do not markedly reduce either the levels of GABA or the activity of its synthetic enzyme L-glutamic acid decarboxylase (GAD) (*McGeer* and *McGeer*, 1975). The fact that lesions do not cause a total loss of nigral GAD (cf. *Lloyd et al.*, 1976) together with results from studies on the behaviour (*Scheel-Kruger et al.*, 1977) and neurophysiology (*Grace* and *Bunney*, 1979) of local injections, it is possible that GABA-utilizing interneurons occur within the substantia nigra, perhaps communicating between the pars reticulata and the pars compacta. The major long GABA-ergic pathway within the EPS initiates in the head of the striatum in laboratory animals (probably both the caudate and putamen in the human) sends collaterals to the globus pallidus and terminates within the substantia nigra (cf. *Fibiger*, 1980). In this latter region the exact distribution of the incoming GABA terminals is not yet determined definitively but it seems very likely that it is to both the pars reticulata neurons and the dopamine (DA) containing cell bodies within the pars compacta. Recent evidence has shown that GABA-ergic neurons either from this striato-nigral path or of an efferent nigral GABA-ergic tract also terminate outside of the substantia nigra, but the exact distribution is still unknown (*Di Chiara et al.*, 1979).

This anatomical distribution of GABA-ergic neurons within the EPS provides for complex neuronal interactions with the major ascending neuronal pathway within the EPS, the nigro-striatal DA system. Thus at least three levels of GABA-DA interactions are possible: (i) within the striatum the GABA-ergic interneurons may terminate on the incoming DA terminals. This is supported by evidence that locally perfused bicuculline or picrotoxin enhances DA release in the cat caudate nucleus: this is reversed by the addition of GABA to the perfusion fluid. GABA itself reduces endogenous DA release *in vivo* (*Bartholini et al.*, 1976). However an indirect effect of GABA on DA release, at the striatal level, may also occur as evidenced by the GABA-induced enhancement of the potassium-stimulated DA release *in vitro* and the increase in formation of DA from its labelled precursor (cf. *Giorguieff et al.* 1977). (ii) The direct inhibition of the DA cell bodies by the striato-nigral GABA-ergic input. Evidence for this is both biochemical (*Bartholini et al.*, 1979 a; *Lloyd*, 1980) and neurophysiological (cf. *Dray* and *Straughan*, 1976). (iii) An indirect excitation of DA neurons at the level of the substantia nigra via the GABA-mediated striato-nigral inhibition of pars reticulata neurons, some of which are possibly inhibitory interneurons tonically controlling the DA cell bodies in the pars compacta (*Cheramy et al.*, 1978; *Grace* and *Bunney*, 1979; *Olianas et al.*, 1978; *Scheel-Kruger et al.*, 1977).

With this admittedly incomplete understanding of the distribution of GABA neurons in the EPS, one can attempt to consider changes in the function of these neurons in disorders of EPS function. These disorders are basically of two different origins-neuropathological, *i.e.* degenerative diseases of the EPS such as Parkinson's disease and Huntington's chorea and iatrogenic, *i.e.* drug-induced, disorders such as L-DOPA or neuroleptic dyskinesias and the neuroleptic-induced Parkinsonism.

B. Alterations of GABA-Ergic Neuron Function in Degenerative Diseases of the EPS

I. Parkinson's Disease

In Parkinson's disease the major neurochemical change is a loss of the nigro-striatal DA pathway, resulting in akinesia and rigidity (*Bernheimer et al.*, 1976; *Hornykiewicz*, 1966; *Lloyd et al.*, 1975). However, the tremor associated with Parkinson's disease does not seem to bear a direct correlation with DA cell loss in the pars compacta (*Bernheimer et al.*, 1973). Other neurochemical changes occur in Parkinson's disease which may be associated with tremor (and also other symptoms). Thus, a substantial loss of noradrenaline and serotonin neurons occurs in the striatum and substantia nigra (cf. *Hornykiewicz*, 1966). However, a large, and perhaps functionally more important, reduction in GABA-ergic neuron activity occurs. This is indicated by a large decrease in GAD activity in all regions of the EPS of non-DOPA treated patients (Table 1). GABA levels themselves are not altered (Table 1). This latter observations may be a result of post-mortem artefacts or possibly reflects that the GABA neurons have not actually degenerated but are in a metabolically depressed state following a prolonged reduction in DA input. This latter hypothesis is supported by the observations that (i) lesion of nigro-striatal DA neurons results in a large decrease in the metabolic activity of the striatum (*Schwartz et al.*, 1976); and (ii) GAD levels of chronically L-DOPA treated patients are relatively "normal" (Table 1). This has been interpreted as indicative of a reversal of a "biochemical atrophy" of GABA-ergic neurons in the untreated Parkinsonian condition, as if GABA-ergic neurons had actually been lost, L-DOPA therapy would not be associated with normalized levels of GAD (cf. *Lloyd*, 1980).

Table 1. *GAD activity, GABA levels and* ³H-GABA *binding in different brain regions from parkinsonian patients*

Brain Region	GAD Levels[a]		GABA Levels	³H-GABA Binding
	No DOPA	L-DOPA treated	No DOPA	All patients
Caudate Nucleus	25.0[b]; 30.8[c]	78.2[b]; 73.1[c]; 101[d]	75.2[e]	107[g]; 94[h]
Putamen	30.3[b]; 50.0[c]	77.5[b]; 75.0[c]; 108.1[d]	103.6[e]	135[g]; 95[h]
Substantia Nigra	20.3[b]; 51.9[c]	95.1[b]; 40.7[c]; 25.9[d]	136.7[f]	31[g]; 54[h]

[a] All values expressed as percent control patients.
Data from: [b] *Lloyd et al.*, 1976; [c] *McGeer et al.*, 1971 (all patients); [d] *Rinne et al.*, 1974; [e] *Hornykiewicz et al.*, 1976; [f] *Perry et al.*, 1973; [g] *Lloyd et al.*, 1977 a; [h] *Rinne et al.*, 1978.

The question of the clinical correlate of these alterations in GAD activity in the EPS is of course of interest. It has been suggested that the decrease in GAD activity in the untreated Parkinsonian condition is a homeostatic manoeuver to maintain the GABA/DA balance in the EPS and that upon reinstatement of the DA tone by chronic L-DOPA therapy the EPS GABA function also returns to normal (cf. *Lloyd*, 1980). However, other interpretations or correlations are also possible. Thus, the tremor of Parkinson's disease is not evidently correlated with the dysfunction of DA neurons, and responds only poorly to acute L-DOPA therapy. Upon prolonged treatment with L-DOPA, the Parkinsonian tremor undergoes a marked amelioration (*Barbeau*, 1969; *Calne* and *Klawans*, 1977), a time-course which has an evident resemblance to that for the L-DOPA-GAD effect. Additional indirect evidence is available for the involvement of striatal GABA neurons in tremor. One of the most efficacious treatments for Parkinsonian tremor is the administration of anticholinergic drugs (*Calne* and *Reid*, 1972; *Greenblatt* and *Shader*, 1973), implying that the excess ACh/DA imbalance in Parkinson's disease is responsible. Increased GABA-ergic tonic (*e.g.* by SL 76 002 or muscimol) effectively diminishes striatal cholinergic activity (*Scatton et al.*, 1980). This may be correlated to the L-DOPA-GAD-antitremor time-course of action.

The above discussion applies to the pathology of GABA neurons, *i.e.* the presynaptic element. Changes in EPS GABA receptors have also been noted in the Parkinsonian condition. In the substantia nigra a loss of 50—75 percent of ³H-GABA binding sites is evident

(Table 1). This is likely at least partially associated with the loss of the DA cell bodies in this region as firstly this latter change is the quantitatively most important morphological and neurochemical alteration to occur in this nucleus (cf. *Hornykiewicz*, 1966; *Lloyd et al.*, 1975), and secondly such a loss in ^{3}H-GABA binding does not occur in the striatum (Table 1) where decreases in serotonin occur similar to those observed in the substantia nigra (cf. *Hornykiewicz*, 1966).

It is of interest to note that the changes observed in GABA neurons in Parkinson's disease have not been reproduced in animal models for this disease. Thus, lesion of the nigro-striatal DA pathway either electrolytically or with 6-OHDA does not alter striatal GAD activity in the cat (*Hockman et al.*, 1971). Similar lesions of the nigro-striatal DA path in the rat produces a reduction in ^{3}H-GABA binding in the hands of some investigators, but not of others (*Gale*, 1980; *Goldstein; Biggio; De Montis;* personal communications). This may indicate that the neuronal connections in the EPS as interpreted from animal models are quite different in the human brain.

II. Huntington's Chorea

This EPS disorder is in many ways a "mirror image" of Parkinson's disease in that the morphological alterations involve a loss of neurons in the striatum whereas the substantia nigra remains pigmented; the patients exhibit hypokinesis and chorea rather akinesia, rigidity and tremor; neurochemically a primary deficit appears to be a loss of GABA neurons (cf. *Enna et al.*, 1977; *Lloyd*, 1980) whereas the relative density of the DA nerve terminals in the striatum is within normal limits (*Bernheimer et al.*, 1973). With regards to the changes in GABA neurons in Huntington's chorea, these are reflected in all aspects of GABA neuron activity (Table 2). GAD activity is severely decreased in the caudate nucleus, putamen, pallidum and substantia nigra. GABA levels themselves are low in the same brain regions and also in the CSF. GABA receptors, as defined by either ^{3}H-GABA or ^{3}H-muscimol binding are severely decreased in the striatum, but not in the substantia nigra (Table 2). This is in contrast to the initial reports that GABA receptors were normal in Huntington's striatum (*Enna et al.*, 1976), however, it is clear from the consistency of the more recent reports that ^{3}H-GABA binding sites are decreased in the striatum of patients with Huntington's chorea.

This alteration of GABA binding sites in the striatum but not in the substantia nigra is consistent with the observation in Huntington's

Table 2. *Indices of GABA synaptic function in post-mortem basal ganglia material from Huntington's chorea patients*

Index of GABA Synaptic function	Caudate Nucleus		Putamen		Substantia Nigra	
	Activity	Reference	Activity	Reference	Activity	Reference
GAD Activity	19	a	19	a		
(percent control	27	b	19	b	31	b
patients)	38	c	32	c		
GABA Levels	43	c	38	d	40	d
(percent control	60	d	41	c		
patients)						
³H-GABA Binding	22	e	25	e	115	g
(percent control	15	g	50	f	106	h
patients)	57	h	56	h		

Data from: a *Stahl* and *Swanson* (1974); b *McGeer* and *McGeer* (1976); c *Bird* and *Iversen* (1974); d *Perry et al.* (1973); e *Lloyd et al.* (1977 b); f *Iversen et al.* (1979); g *Olsen et al.* (1979); h *Reisine et al.* (1979).

chorea of a massive neuronal degeneration in the striatum whereas the substantia nigra is relatively spared. These alterations in GABA receptors may be important for the pharmacotherapy of Huntington's chorea. From the parallelism of the changes in GABA neuron function in Huntington's chorea and DA neuron changes in Parkinson's disease, it could be expected that GABA replacement therapy would be efficacious in HC (cf. *Bartholini* this supplement for discussion). However, such replacement therapy will depend on the presence of GABA receptors. As these are decreased in the Huntington's striatum, it seems that the only hope for GABA replacement therapy in the striatum is that the remaining receptors are supersensitive to GABA or the therapeutically administered GABA mimetic. Using the cerebellar cortex from HC patients as a model for striatal changes (as the latter structure does not have sufficient tissue remaining to perform experiments) it has been shown that the K_d for GABA binding in the Huntington's brain is considerably lower than controls (30 nm versus 120 nm for non-Triton-X-100 treated membranes) indicating that the binding site has a higher affinity for GABA (cf. *Lloyd*, 1980). It is possible that this is related to an alteration in membrane phospholipids as Triton-X-100 and phospholipase C, which normally increase the affinity of ³H-GABA binding in HC cerebellar, do not alter ³H-GABA binding to cerebellar membranes from HC patients (*Lloyd* and *Davidson*, 1979). In this context it is of interest to note that the concentration of both phosphoethanolamine and glycerophosphoethanolamine are abnormal in HC brains (*Perry et al.,* 1973) and that these substances, which are derived from membrane phospholipids, apparently alter GABA receptor function (*Watkins,* 1966; *Giambalvo* and *Rosengren,* 1976; *Johnston* and *Kennedy,* 1978).

C. GABA Neuron Function in Drug-Induced EPS Disorders

I. Drug-Induced Parkinsonism

In terms of the human condition, the author is not aware of any post-mortem studies which clearly relate to the function of GABA systems; therefore the only inferences that can be made are those obtained by the study of animal models. Thus, neuroleptic drugs which induce a Parkinsonian syndrome in man produce a state of catalepsy in the laboratory rat. In relation to this, the cataleptogenic neuroleptics acutely lower GABA levels in the striatum and substantia nigra whereas "silent" neuroleptics (devoid of a cataleptogenic effect) do not produce such a decrease (*Lloyd* and *Hornykiewicz,* 1977). Furthermore, the co-administration of a GABA agonist with a cataleptogenic (but not a "silent") neuroleptic greatly enhances the induction of catalepsy (cf. *Lloyd,* 1980). Upon chronic (weeks—months) administration of a neuroleptic, there is a large degree of tolerance to the cataleptogenic effect (cf. *Lloyd* and *Worms,* 1980 for refs.). In parallel with this is the tolerance to the neuroleptic-induced changes in GABA levels in the substantia nigra (*Lloyd* and *Hornykiewicz,* 1977). Furthermore, co-administration of a GABA agonist with the neuroleptic blocks the development of tolerance (*Lloyd* and *Worms,* 1980). Taken together these observations can be interpreted as indicating that in a cataleptic state the GABA system undergoes changes in order to minimize the catalepsy; as the system returns to normal (*i.e.* tolerance develops) the GABA system also returns to normal. However, if the GABA input is maintained (*e.g.* by a GABA agonist) then the degree of catalepsy is enhanced and the development of tolerance is inhibited. This implies that GABA mimetics are to be avoided in the treatment of drug induced Parkinsonism, but that non-toxic GABA antagonists may play a role in these EPS disorders.

II. Drug-Induced Dyskinesias

As for the problem of drug-induced Parkinsonism (see above) nothing is known about post-mortem EPS alterations in GABA function in the human condition (*i.e.* tardive dyskinesias induced by L-DOPA or neuroleptics). Furthermore, animal models are usually indirect—*i.e.* the supersensitivity to apomorphine (or other DA mimetics) after withdrawal from prolonged neuroleptic administration is studied rather than the direct induction of stereotypies by DA mimetics or neuroleptics. In this type of model, co-administration of a GABA agonist with the neuroleptic largely blocks the supersensitivity to the stereotypic effect of apomorphine (*Lloyd* and *Worms*, 1980). Acutely haloperidol decreases ^{3}H-GABA binding in the cerebellum or striatum (*Lloyd et al.*, 1977 c; *Trabucchi et al.*, 1978). Upon chronic (6-month) administration this alteration is maintained (*Lloyd et al.*, 1977 c). Although L-DOPA does not induce stereotypies over a 6-month administration period in rats, the initially elevated GABA levels in the substantia nigra are normal at the end of the treatment period (*Lloyd* and *Hornykiewicz*, 1977). This indicates that upon chronic L-DOPA administration (which induces stereotypies in man) there is a modulation of EPS GABA neuron function. Together with the blockade of apomorphine-induced stereotyped behaviour by GABA mimetics (cf. *Lloyd*, 1980), the above evidence indicates that the control of stereotypies associated with excessive DA receptor activation may be susceptible to control by GABA agonist therapy. Preliminary clinical trials with SL 76 002 (*Bartholini et al.*, 1979 b) support this hypothesis.

References

Barbeau, A.: L-DOPA therapy in Parkinson's disease: a critical review of nine year's experience. Canad. Med. Assoc. J. *101*, 59—68 (1969).

Bartholini, G., Stadler, H., Gadea-Ciria, M., Lloyd, K. G.: The use of the push-pull cannulla to estimate the dynamics of acetylcholine and catecholamines within various brain areas. Neuropharmacology *15*, 515—519 (1976).

Bartholini, G., Scatton, B., Zivkovic, B., Lloyd, K. G.: On the mode of action of SL 76 002, a new GABA receptor agonist. In: GABA-Neurotransmitters, pp. 326—339. Copenhagen: Munksgaard. 1979 a.

Bartholini, G., Lloyd, K. G., Worms, P., Constantinidis, J., Tissot, R.: GABA and GABA-ergic medication: relation to striatal dopamine function and Parkinsonism. In: Parkinson's Disease, pp. 253—257. New York: Raven Press. 1979 b.

Bernheimer, H., Birkmayer, W., Hornykiewicz, O., Jellinger, K., Seitelberger, F.: Brain dopamine and the syndroms of Parkinson and Huntington. J. Neurol. Sci. *20*, 415—455 (1973).

Bird, E. D., Iversen, L. L.: Huntington's chorea: post-mortem measurement of glutamic acid decarboxylase, choline acetylase and dopamine in basal ganglia. Brain *97*, 457—472 (1974).

Calne, D. B., Klawans, H. L.: Pathophysiology and pharmacotherapy of tremor. Pharmacol. Therap. C. 2, 113—123 (1977).

Calne, D. B., Reid, J. L.: Antiparkinsonian drugs: pharmacological and therapeutic aspects. Drugs 4, 49—74 (1972).

Cheramy, A., Nieoullon, A., Glowinski, J.: Role of GABA-ergic and glycinergic transmission in the substantia nigra in the regulation of dopamine release in the cat caudate nucleus. In: Amino Acids as Chemical Transmitters, pp. 413—423. New York: Plenum. 1978.

Di Chiara, G., Proceddu, M. L., Morselli, M., Mulas, M. L., Gessa, G. L.: Strio-nigral and nigro-thalamic GABA-ergic neurons as output paths for striatal responses. In: GABA-Neurotransmitters, pp. 465—481. Copenhagen: Munksgaard. 1979.

Dray, A., Straughan, D. W.: Synaptic mechanisms in the substantia nigra. J. Pharm. Pharmacol. 28, 400—405 (1976).

Enna, S. J., Bennett, J. P., Bylund, D. B., Snyder, S. H., Bird, E. D., Iversen, L. L.: Alteration of brain neurotransmitter binding in Huntington's chorea. Brain Res. 116, 531—537 (1976).

Enna, S. J., Stern, L. Z., Wastek, G. J., Yamamura, H. I.: Minireview: Neurobiology and pharmacology of Huntington's disease. Life Sci. 20, 205—212 (1977).

Fibiger, H. C.: Organization and plasticity of GABA-ergic neurons in extrapyramidal and limbic structures of the rat. In: GABA and Other Inhibitory Transmitters. Fayetteville: Ankho. 1980 (in press).

Gale, K.: GABA receptor binding in substantia nigra: alterations induced by surgical and chemical lesions. In: GABA and Other Inhibitory Neurotransmitters. Fayetteville: Ankho. 1980 (in press).

Giambalvo, C., Rosengren, P.: The effect of phospholipases and proteases on the binding of γ-aminobutyric acid to junctional complexes of rat cerebellum. Biochem. Biophys. Acta 436, 741—756 (1976).

Giorguieff, M. F., Kemel, M. L., Besson, M. J., Glowinski, G.: Involvement of cholinergic and GABA-receptors in the control of dopamine release from rat striatal slices. In: Parkinson's Disease: Concepts and Prospects, pp. 31—42. Amsterdam: Excerpta Medica. 1977.

Grace, A. A., Bunney, B. S.: Paradoxical GABA excitation of nigral dopaminergic cells: indirect medication through reticulata inhibitory neurons. Europ. J. Pharmacol. 59, 211—218 (1979).

Greenblatt, D. L., Shader, R. I.: Anticholinergics. New Engl. J. Med. 288, 1215—1219 (1973).

Hockman, C. H., Lloyd, K. G., Farley, I. J., Hornykiewicz, O.: Experimental midbrain lesions: neurochemical comparison between the animal model and Parkinson's disease. Brain Res. 35, 613—618 (1971).

Hornykiewicz, O.: Dopamine (3-hydroxytyramine) and brain function. Pharmacol. Revs 18, 925—964 (1966).

Hornykiewicz, O., Lloyd, K. G., Davidson, L.: The GABA system, function of the basal ganglia, and Parkinson's disease. In: GABA in Nervous System Function, pp. 479—485. New York: Raven Press. 1976.

Iversen, L. L., Bird, E. D., Spokes, E., Nicholson, S. H., Suckling, C. J.: Agonist specificity of GABA binding sites in human brain and GABA in Huntington's disease and schizophrenia. In: GABA-Neurotransmitters, pp. 179—190. Copenhagen: Munksgaard. 1979.

Johnston, G. A. R., Kennedy, S. M.: GABA receptors and phospholipids. In: Amino Acids as Chemical Transmitters, pp. 507—516. New York: Plenum. 1978.

Lloyd, K. G.: Indications for GABA neuron dysfunction in mental disease. In: Enzymes and Neurotransmitters in Mental Disease. New York: Raven Press. 1980 (in press).

Lloyd, K. G., Davidson, L.: (^{3}H)GABA binding in brains from Huntington's chorea patients: altered regulation by phospholipids? Science 205, 1147 to 1149 (1979).

Lloyd, K. G., Hornykiewicz, O.: Effect of chronic neuroleptic or L-DOPA administration on GABA levels in the rat substantia nigra. Life Sci. 21, 1489—1496 (1977).

Lloyd, K. G., Worms, P.: Sustained gamma-aminobutyric acid receptor stimulation and chronic neuroleptic effects. In: Long-Term Effects of Neuroleptics. New York: Raven Press. 1980 (in press).

Lloyd, K. G., Davidson, L., Hornykiewicz, O.: The neurochemistry of Parkinson's disease: effect of L-DOPA therapy. J. Pharmacol. Exp. Therap. 195, 453—464 (1975).

Lloyd, K. G., Möhler, H., Bartholini, G., Hornykiewicz, O.: Pathological alterations in glutamic acid decarboxylase activity in Parkinson's disease. In: Advances in Parkinsonism, pp. 186—192. Basle: Editiones Roche. 1976.

Lloyd, K. G., Shemen, L., Hornykiewicz, O.: Distribution of high affinity sodium-independent (^{3}H)-gamma-aminobutyric acid binding in the human brain: alterations in Parkinson's disease. Brain Res. 127, 269 to 278 (1977 a).

Lloyd, K. G., Dreksler, S., Bird, E. D.: Alterations in ^{3}H-GABA binding in Huntington's chorea. Life Sci. 21, 747—754 (1977 b).

Lloyd, K. G., Shibuya, M., Davidson, L., Hornykiewicz, O.: Chronic neuroleptic therapy: tolerance and GABA systems. In: Non-striatal Dopamine Neurons, pp. 409—415. New York: Raven Press. 1977 c.

McGeer, P. L., McGeer, E. G.: Evidence for glutamic acid decarboxylase-containing interneurons in the neostriatum. Brain Res. 91, 331—335 (1975).

McGeer, P. L., McGeer, E. G.: The GABA system and function of the basal ganglia: Huntington's disease. In: GABA in Nervous System Function, pp. 487—495. New York: Raven Press. 1976.

McGeer, P. L., McGeer, E. G., Wada, J. A.: Glutamic acid decarboxylase in Parkinson's disease and epilepsy. Neurology 21, 1000—1007 (1971).

Olianas, M. C., De Montis, G. M., Mulas, G., Tagliamonte, A.: The striatal dopaminergic function is mediated by the inhibition of a nigral non-dopaminergic neuronal system via a striato-nigral GABA-ergic pathway. Europ. J. Pharmacol. 49, 223—232 (1978).

Olsen, R. W., Van Ness, P. C., Tourtellotte, W. W.: Gamma-aminobutyric acid receptor binding curves for human brain regions: comparison of Huntington's disease and normal. In: Huntington's Disease, pp. 697 to 704. New York: Raven Press. 1979.

Perry, T. L., Hansen, S., Kloster, M.: Huntington's chorea: deficiency of γ-aminobutyric acid in brain. New Engl. J. Med. *288*, 337—342 (1973).

Reisine, T. D., Beaumont, K., Bird, E. D., Spokes, E., Yamamura, H. I.: Huntington's disease: alterations in neurotransmitter receptor binding in the human brain. In: Huntington's Disease, pp. 717—726. New York: Raven Press. 1979.

Rinne, U. K., Sonninen, V., Riekkinen, P., Laaksonen, H.: Dopaminergic nervous transmission in Parkinson's disease. Med. Biol. *52*, 208—217 (1974).

Rinne, U. K., Koskinen, V., Laaksonen, H., Lönnenberg, P., Sonninen, V.: GABA receptor binding in the Parkinsonian brain. Life Sci. *22*, 2225 to 2228 (1978).

Scatton, B., Bartholini, G.: Modulation by GABA of cholinergic transmission in rat brain. In: GABA and Other Inhibitory Neurotransmitters. Fayetteville: Ankho. 1980 (in press).

Scheel-Kruger, J., Arnt, J., Magelund, G.: Behavioural stimulation induced by muscimol and other GABA agonists injected into the substantia nigra. Neurosci. Letts *4*, 351—356 (1977).

Schwartz, W. J., Sharp, F. R., Gunn, R. H., Evarts, E. V.: Lesions of ascending dopaminergic pathways decrease forebrain glucose uptake. Nature *261*, 155—157 (1976).

Stahl, W. L., Swanson, P. D.: Biochemical abnormalities in Huntington's chorea. Neurology *24*, 813—819 (1974).

Watkins, J. C.: Pharmacological receptors and general permeability of cell membranes. J. Theoret. Biol. *9*, 37—50 (1965).

Author's address: Dr. *K. G. Lloyd*, Department of Neuropharmacology, Synthélabo–L.E.R.S., 31, av. P. V. Couturier, F-92220 Bagneux, France.

Journal of Neural Transmission, Suppl. 16, 229—238 (1980)

The Potential of GABA-Mimetics in the Therapy of Extrapyramidal Disorders

G. Bartholini and K. G. Lloyd

Research Department, Synthélabo–L.E.R.S., Paris, France

Summary

GABA mimetics inhibit extrapyramidal DA and ACh neurons and affect an unknown system beyond both DA and ACh receptors, which is involved in extrapyramidal motor outputs. Based on these data, the rationale is discussed for the clinical use of GABA mimetics in Huntington's chorea, parkinsonian tremor, L-DOPA or neuroleptic-induced dyskinesias.

I. Introduction

GABA mimetics represent a new class of potential drugs for disorders of the extrapyramidal system. This view is based on the role exerted by GABA in the basal ganglia as evidenced by experimental data as well as by clinical results with compounds which affect GABA-ergic transmission. This article focusses upon (a) the sites of action of GABA mimetics on the basal ganglia neuronal network, (b) the alterations of GABA neurons in extrapyramidal disorders, and (c) the rationale for the clinical use of GABA mimetics.

For the therapeutic potentials of these drugs in other pathological states such as epilepsy, spasticity, schizophrenia and affective disorders, the reader is referred to *Lloyd* (1980) and *Morselli et al.* (1980).

II. Sites of Action of GABA-Mimetics Within the Extrapyramidal Systems

The date discussed in the following has been mainly obtained by using two GABA mimetics, muscimol and SL 76 002.

Muscimol is GABA in a cyclized configuration. The compound is one of the most active GABA receptor agonists as determined by displacing ^{3}H-GABA from binding sites of brain membrane preparations (*Enna* and *Snyder*, 1975; *Lloyd* and *Dreksler*, 1979). It poorly crosses the blood-brain barrier and is rapidly metabolized (*Baraldi et al.*, 1975; *Maggi* and *Enna*, 1979). In humans, muscimol causes hallucinations and confusional states (*Chase* and *Tamminga*, 1975).

SL 76 002[1], 4-[2′-hydroxy-4′-fluoro-α-(4″-chlorophenyl)benzene-methanimino]butyramide, a derivative of a substituted benzophenone and GABAMIDE, is a GABA-agonist as indicated by electrophysiological experiments (*Desarmenien et al.*, 1980; *Lloyd et al.*, 1979 a).

In mammals, this compound readily enters the brain and is metabolized to GABA receptor stimulants (including GABA itself). SL 76 002 and its metabolites displace GABA from binding sites. The compound does not modify other biochemical parameters in the brain related to GABA neuron function (*Bartholini et al.*, 1979 a) and thus can be considered an apparently pure GABA receptor agonist. Due to its characteristics and the apparent lack of toxicity, SL 76 002 is undergoing clinical trials in neuropsychiatric patients (see below).

Both muscimol and SL 76 002 have at least three sites of action in the extrapyramidal system:

A. Dopaminergic Neurons

Dopaminergic neurons are inhibited by GABA mimetics which probably act on receptors located on both dopamine (DA) cell bodies and terminals (cf. *Bartholini et al.*, 1976; *Lloyd et al.*, 1977 a). This is evidenced by the decrease in DA synthesis and release (*Bartholini et al.*, 1979 a, b) and by the potentiation by GABA mimetics of the behavioural effect of neuroleptic drugs (catalepsy; *Lloyd et al.*, 1979 a): thus, reduction in DA liberation further augments the effect of the DA receptor blockade by neuroleptics. This action of GABA mimetics is exerted at doses similar to those necessary for reducing DA turnover (100—200 mg/kg i.p. for SL 76 002 and 2—5 mg/kg i.p. for muscimol, cf. *Lloyd et al.*, 1980).

B. Cholinergic Neurons

Striatal cholinergic neurons are inhibited by GABA mimetics as reflected by the accumulation of striatal acetylcholine (ACh) due to

---

[1] Synthetized by Dr. J. P. Kaplan, Chemistry Department, Synthélabo-L.E.R.S., Paris.

diminished release of the transmitter (*Scatton* and *Bartholini*, 1980). This effect occurs at threshold doses of GABA mimetics lower than those affecting the DA system: thus, SL 76 002 and muscimol show a significant effect on ACh levels at dose as low as 50 and 0.2 mg/kg i.p., respectively (*Scatton* and *Bartholini*, 1980). Behaviourally, this action probably results in facilitation of the striatal control of muscle tone and motility as such low doses of GABA mimetics antagonize the neuroleptic-induced catalepsy (*Worms* and *Lloyd*, 1980) and potentiate the stereotyped behaviour caused by apomorphine (*Worms* and *Lloyd*, unpublished results). This may be explained by the observation that, inter-alia, striatal cholinergic neurons exert a key role in determining extrapyramidal function, for instance by translating the changes of dopaminergic transmission into motor outputs (*Bartholini et al.*, 1976).

C. Unknown Neurons Postsynaptic to DA and ACh Systems

1. Acute GABA Mimetic Administration

Changes in dopaminergic transmission are not only mediated by cholinergic neurons. Thus, the apomorphine-induced stereotypies are blocked by GABA mimetics (*Bartholini et al.*, 1979 b) and this is independent of the action of these drugs on both DA neurons (which are not involved in the apomorphine effect) and cholinergic neurons (the depression of which results in potentiation of apomorphine). Therefore, as a working hypothesis, it can be assumed that GABA receptors inhibit a system postsynaptic to both DA and ACh neurons, which is sensitive to apomorphine. The nature and the location of this target is presently unknown.

2. Repeated GABA Mimetic Administration

The existence of such a mechanism is also supported by the influence of GABA mimetics on long-term effects of neuroleptics: increase in GABA-ergic transmission affects the changes in sensitivity to DA of target system(s) of dopaminergic neurons: thus, the supersensitivity which develops following repeated neuroleptic treatment—as evidenced by the increase in the threshold dose of apomorphine for eliciting stereotypies and by the reduction of the cataleptogenic action of neuroleptics—is antagonized by co-administration of GABA mimetics (*Lloyd* and *Worms*, 1980). This effect is independent of changes in DA and ACh neuron activity: thus, these neurons during repeated treatment with GABA mimetics develop tolerance to the acute action of these drugs (unpublished results). This indicates that the neuronal set-up which is involved in development of supersensitivity of DA target system and which is affected by GABA mimetics is postsynaptic to both DA and ACh neurons.

Table 1 summarizes the actions of GABA mimetics in the extra-pyramidal system.

Table 1. *GABA mimetics and extrapyramidal system*

Site of action	Action	Effect	Potential therapeutic indication
DA neurons	Inhibitory	Potentiation of neuroleptic-induced catelepsy	Huntington's chorea Neuroleptic-induced tardive dyskinesias
ACh neurons	Inhibitory	Antagonism of neuroleptic-induced catalepsy Potentiation of apomorphine-induced stereotypies	Parkinsonian tremor?
Unknown neurons	?	Antagonism of apomorphine-induced stereotypies Antagonism of the tolerance to chronic neuroleptic treatment	L-DOPA-induced involuntary movements Huntington's chorea Neuroleptic-induced tardive dyskinesias

III. Disorders of the Extrapyramidal System. Therapeutic Potential of GABA Mimetics

Disorders of the experimental system are determined by either primary degenerative processes or drugs. In both cases, it appears that GABA neurons are involved.

A. Degenerative Disorders

1. Parkinson's Disease

In the extrapyramidal system of non-L-DOPA treated par-kinsonian patients, beside the reduction of biochemical parameters related to DA neurons (*Lloyd et al.*, 1975; *Hornykiewicz*, 1966) and the loss of the DA cell bodies in the pars compacta of the substantia nigra (cf. *Bernheimer et al.*, 1973), there is severe decrease (75—80 %) of glutamic acid decarboxylase activity in the striatum and substantia nigra (cf. *Lloyd*, 1980). The loss of DA neurons is correlated with the severity of akinesia and rigidity (*Bernheimer et al.*, 1973) and L-DOPA therapy is of marked benefit for these symptoms (*Barbeau*,

1969; *Calne* and *Reid*, 1972). However, the severity of the tremor in Parkinson's disease does not appear to be correlated with DA neuron loss (*Bernheimer et al.*, 1973). Thus, this symptom is ameliorated by long-term L-DOPA (*Barbeau*, 1969; *Calne* and *Klawans*, 1977) therapy which also results in a less marked diminution of glutamic acid decarboxylase activity in extrapyramidal centers (*Lloyd* and *Hornykiewicz*, 1973). This has been interpreted as indicating that reduction of dopaminergic transmission results in a "biochemical atrophy" of GABA neurons which, upon chronic L-DOPA therapy, gradually regain their activity (*Lloyd* and *Hornykiewicz*, 1973). This is supported by the observation that destruction of the nigrostriatal DA path markedly lowers the metabolic activity of the striatum, as evidenced by measuring the utilization of $2\text{-}^{14}C$ deoxyglucose (*Schwartz et al.*, 1976).

According to these findings, and based on the inhibitory influence of GABA mimetics on striatal cholinergic neurons (see section II B), it might be assumed that low doses of these compounds are useful in the treatment of parkinsonian patients with pronounced tremor. This is also supported by the anti-tremor action of anticholinergic drugs in Parkinson's disease (*Calne* and *Reid*, 1972; *Greenblatt* and *Shader*, 1973). However, it should be noted that in cases of Parkinson's disease with marked rigidity and/or akinesia, GABA mimetics have to be avoided as such drugs (at least in high doses) decrease the activity of DA neurons (see section II A).

2. Huntington's Chorea

The neuropathology and symptomatology of Huntington's chorea is considered as the "mirror image" of Parkinson's disease, with striatal neuron loss, but intact substantia nigra and chorea and athetosis rather than akinesia and rigidity. There appears to be a primary degeneration of GABA neurons in the extrapyramidal system (cf. *Enna et al.*, 1977; *Lloyd*, 1980) which probably triggers a relative increase in dopaminergic transmission due to the diminution of the inhibitory GABA input on DA neurons. In such a situation, replacement therapy by GABA agonists or their precursors should be of beneficial effect due to their inhibitory action on DA neurons. Such an assumption is supported by the observation that GABA mimetics enhance the cataleptogenic action of neuroleptics in the rat (see section II A), and reduce the extrapyramidal symptoms in Huntington's chorea (*Bartholini et al.*, 1979 a). Most clinical studies with GABA mimetics, however, has provided negative results. Thus muscimol, up to toxic levels, is ineffective (*Chase* and *Tamminga*, 1975). Similarly, GABA-transaminase inhibitors such as γ-acetylenic

GABA (*Y. Agid,* personal communication) or aminooxyacetic acid (*T. L. Perry,* personal communication) fail to ameliorate the symptoms of Huntington's chorea. Two GABA-mimetic compounds have, however, shown some degree of therapeutic success in this disease: isoniazid (a non-specific GABA-transaminase inhibitor, *Perry et al.,* 1978) and SL 76 002 (*Morselli et al.,* 1980).

A likely reason for the fact that GABA mimetics are effective only in some cases of Huntington's chorea is that, in this disease, not only have the GABA neurons degenerated but also there is a large loss of GABA receptors in the striatum. Evidence for this is provided by the decrease in ^{3}H-GABA or ^{3}H-muscimol binding sites of membranes prepared from the caudate nucleus or putamen of Huntington's chorea patients (*Iversen et al.,* 1979; *Lloyd et al.,* 1977 b; *Olsen et al.,* 1979; *Reisine et al.,* 1979). The positive response of some patients to GABA-mimetic therapy may be due to (a) a possibly less severe loss of GABA receptors in the early stage of the disease (*Bartholini et al.,* 1979 a) and/or (b) a supersensitivity of the remaining GABA receptors. Such a supersensitivity has been demonstrated in the cerebellum (*Lloyd* and *Davidson,* 1979) and cerebral cortex (*Lloyd* and *Ziegler,* unpublished) of brains from Huntington's chorea patients.

B. Drug-Induced Disorders

1. L-DOPA-Induced Dyskinesias

One of the severe side-effects of L-DOPA therapy in Parkinson's disease is the development of abnormal involuntary movements which is probably connected with an excessive formation and liberation of DA (cf. *Barbeau,* 1976). In animal models, the equivalent of this side-effect (apomorphine-induced stereotyped behaviour in rats) is ameliorated by GABA mimetics (*e.g.* SL 76 002, muscimol, see section II B) (*Lloyd et al.,* 1980). Accordingly, these drugs may have a therapeutic action on dyskinesias induced by L-DOPA in parkinsonian patients. Indeed, this view appears to be supported by preliminary results with SL 76 002 (*Morselli et al.,* 1980; *Bartholini et al.,* 1979 b).

2. Neuroleptic-Induced Tardive Dyskinesias

The tardive dyskinesias induced by chronic neuroleptic administration is a severe and frequent side-effect in the treatment of schizophrenia. The development of the dyskinesias is likely due to supersensitivity of target system(s) of DA neurons (cf. *Tarsy* and *Baldessarini,* 1977). The fact that GABA mimetics decrease the tolerance to the cataleptogenic action of neuroleptics and enhance the threshold dose of apomorphine for inducing stereotypies (see section II C) suggests that GABA is involved in the development of supersensitivity. Accordingly, GABA receptor agonists should prevent tardive dyskinesias. Finally, this syndrome may be ameliorated by GABA mimetics via their inhibitory action on DA neurons (see section II A). Preliminary clinical observations with muscimol (*Chase* and *Tamminga*, 1979) or SL 76 002 (*Morselli et al.*, 1980) support this view.

3. Neuroleptic-Induced Parkinsonism

As stated above and according to several authors (*e.g. Kaariainen*, 1976; *Keller et al.*, 1976; *Lloyd et al.*, 1979) diverse GABA mimetics (muscimol, SL 76 002, aminooxyacetic acid, etc.) exacerbate neuroleptic-induced catalepsy. This, however, occurs with doses of GABA mimetics which decrease DA turnover. Smaller doses which apparently only reduce the activity of the cholinergic system should theoretically be useful in the treatment of rigidity and tremor. These latter symptoms in fact are associated with a cholinergic hyperactivity as they are ameliorated by anti-ACh drugs (*Greenblatt* and *Shader*, 1973). (In contrast, hypokinesia does not have a cholinergic component being improved only by L-DOPA.) No information is available on the effect of GABA mimetics in parkinsonism. Some preliminary results indicate that low doses of SL 76 002 improves L-DOPA-induced dyskinesias in Parkinson's disease without aggravating parkinsonian symptoms (*Bartholini et al.*, 1979 b) (see section III B1). However, due to the inhibitory action of GABA mimetics on DA neurons, even if at doses higher than those affecting the cholinergic system, it would seem prudent to avoid the association neuroleptic-GABA mimetic in cases of neuroleptic-induced parkinsonism.

Table 1 summarizes the potential therapeutic indications of GABA mimetics in extrapyramidal disorders.

References

Baraldi, M., Grandison, L., Guidotti, A.: Distribution and metabolism of muscimol in the brain and other tissues of the rat. Neuropharmacology *18*, 57—62 (1979).

Barbeau, A.: L-DOPA therapy in Parkinson's disease: a critical review of nine years' experience. Canad. Med. Assoc. J. *101*, 59—68 (1969).

Barbeau, A.: Neurological and psychiatric side-effects of L-DOPA. Pharmacol. Therap. C *1*, 475—494 (1976).

Bartholini, G., Stadler, H., Gadea-Ciria, M., Lloyd, K. G.: The use of the push-pull cannula to estimate the dynamus of acetylcholine and catecholamines within various brain areas. Neuropharmacology *15*, 515—519 (1976).

Bartholini, G., Scatton, B., Zivkovic, B., Lloyd, K. G.: On the mode of action of SL 76 002, a new GABA receptor agonist. In: GABA-Neurotransmitters, pp. 326—339. Copenhagen: Munksgaard. 1979 a.

Bartholini, G., Lloyd, K. G., Worms, P., Constantinidis, J., Tissot, R.: GABA and GABA-ergic medication: relation to striatal dopamine function and parkinsonism. In: Advances in Neurology, Vol. 24, pp. 253 to 257. New York: Raven Press. 1979 b.

Bernheimer, H., Birkmayer, W., Hornykiewicz, O., Jellinger, K., Seitelberger, F.: Brain dopamine and the syndroms of Parkinson and Huntington. J. Neurol. Sci. 20, 415—455 (1973).

Calne, D. B., Klawans, H. L.: Pathophysiology and pharmacotherapy of tremor. Pharmacol. Therap. C 2, 113—123 (1977).

Calne, D. B., Reid, J. L.: Antiparkinsonian drugs: pharmacological and therapeutic aspects. Drugs *4*, 49—72 (1972).

Chase, T. N., Tamminga, C. A.: GABA system participation in human motor, cognitive and neuroendocrine function. In: GABA-Neurotransmitters, pp. 283—294. Copenhagen: Munksgaard. 1979.

Desarmenien, M., Feltz, P., Headley, P. M., Santangelo, F.: Effects of various GABA-mimetics on dorsal ganglion (DRG) neurons: a neurophysiological analysis. In: GABA and Other Inhibitory Neurotransmitters. Fayetteville: Ankho. 1980 (in press).

Enna, S. J., Snyder, S. H.: Properties of γ-aminobutyric acid (GABA) receptor binding in rat brain synaptic membrane fractions. Brain Res. *100*, 81—97 (1975).

Enna, S. J., Stern, L. Z., Wastek, G. J., Yamamura, H. L.: Minireview: Neurobiology and pharmacology of Huntington's disease. Life Sci. 20, 205—212 (1977).

Greenblatt, D. L., Shader, R. I.: Anticholinergics. New Engl. J. Med. *288*, 1215—1219 (1973).

Hornykiewicz, O.: Dopamine (3-hydroxytyramine) and brain function. Pharmacol. Revs *18*, 925—964 (1966).

Iversen, L. L., Bird, E. D., Spokes, E., Nicholson, S. H., Suckling, C. J.: Agonist specifity of GABA binding sites in human brain and GABA in Huntington's disease and schizophrenia. In: GABA-Neurotransmitters, pp. 179—190. Copenhagen: Munksgaard. 1979.

Kaariainen, I.: Effect of aminooxyacetic acid and baclofen on the catalepsy and on the increase of mesolimbic and striatal dopamine turnover induced by haloperidol in rats. Acta Pharmacol. Toxicol. *39*, 393—400 (1976).

Keller, H. H., Schaffner, R., Haefely, W.: Interaction of benzodiazepines with neuroleptics at central dopamine neurons. Naunyn-Schmiedeberg's Arch. Pharmacol. *294*, 1—4 (1976).

Lloyd, K. G.: Indications for GABA neuron dysfunction in mental disease. In: Enzymes and Neurotransmitters in Mental Disease. New York: Raven Press. 1980 (in press).

Lloyd, K. G., Davidson, L.: [³H]GABA binding in brains from Huntington's chorea patients: altered regulation by phospholipids. Science *205*, 1147—1149 (1979).

Lloyd, K. G., Dreksler, S.: An analysis of [³H]Gamma-aminobutyric acid (GABA) binding in the human brain. Brain Res. *163*, 77—87 (1979).

Lloyd, K. G., Hornykiewicz, O.: L-glutamic acid decarboxylase in Parkinson's disease: effect of L-DOPA therapy. Nature *243*, 521—523 (1973).

Lloyd, K. G., Worms, P.: Sustained gamma-aminobutyric acid receptor stimulation and chronic neuroleptic effects. In: Long-Term Effects of Neuroleptics. New York: Raven Press. 1980 (in press).

Lloyd, K. G., Davidson, L., Hornykiewicz, O.: The neurochemistry of Parkinson's disease: effect of L-DOPA therapy. J. Pharmacol. Exp. Therap. *195*, 453—464 (1975).

Lloyd, K. G., Shemen, L., Hornykiewicz, O.: Distribution of high affinity sodium-independent (³H)gamma-aminobutyric acid (³H-GABA) binding in the human brain: alterations in Parkinson's disease. Brain Res. *127*, 269—278 (1977 a).

Lloyd, K. G., Dreksler, S., Bird, E. D.: Alterations in ³H-GABA binding in Huntington's chorea. Life Sci. *21*, 747—754 (1977 b).

Lloyd, K. G., Worms, P., Depoortere, H., Bartholini, G.: Pharmacological profile of SL 76 002, a new GABA mimetic drug. In: GABA-Neurotransmitters, pp. 308—325. Copenhagen: Munksgaard. 1979.

Lloyd, K. G., Worms, P., Zivkovic, B., Scatton, B., Bartholini, G.: Interaction of GABA mimetics with nigro-striatal dopamine neurons. In: GABA and Other Inhibitory Transmitters. Fayetteville: Ankho. 1980 (in press).

Maggi, A., Enna, S. J.: Characteristics of muscimol accumulation in mouse brain after systemic administration. Neuropharmacology *18*, 361—366 (1979).

Morselli, P. L., Bossi, L., Henry, J. P., Zarifian, E., Bartholini, G.: On the therapeutic action of SL 76 002, a new GABA mimetic agents: preliminary observations in neuropsychiatric disorders. In: GABA and Other Inhibitory Neurotransmitters. Fayetteville: Ankho. 1980 (in press).

Olsen, R. W., Wan Ness, P. C., Tourtelotte, W. W.: Gamma-aminobutyric acid receptor binding curves for human brain regions: comparison of Huntington's disease and normal. In: Huntington's Disease, pp. 697 to 704. New York: Raven Press. 1979.

Perry, T. L., Mac Leod, P. M., Hansen, S.: Treatment of Huntington's chorea with isoniazid. New Engl. J. Med. *297*, 840 (1977).

Reisine, T. D., Beaumont, K., Bird, E. D., Spokes, E., Yamamura, H. I.: Huntington's disease: alterations in neurotransmitter receptor binding in the human brain. In: Huntington's Disease, pp. 717—726. New York: Raven Press. 1979.

Scatton, B., Bartholini, G.: Modulation of cholinergic transmission in the rat brain by GABA mimetics. In: GABA and Other Inhibitory Transmitters. Fayetteville: Ankho. 1980 (in press).

Schwartz, W. J., Sharp, F. R., Gunn, R. H., Evarts, E. V.: Lesions of ascending dopaminergic pathways decrease forebrain glucose uptake. Nature *261,* 155—157 (1976).

Tarsy, D., Baldessarini, R. J.: The pathophysiologic basis of tardive dyskinesia. Biol. Psychiat. *12,* 431—450 (1977).

Worms, P., Lloyd, K. G.: Biphasic effects of direct, but not indirect, GABA mimetics and antagonists on haloperidol-induced catalepsy. Naunyn-Schmiedeberg's Arch. Pharmacol. 1980 (in press).

Authors' address: Dr. *G. Bartholini,* Research Department, Synthélabo–L.E.R.S., 58, rue de la Glacière, F-75013 Paris, France.

Subject Index